WHOLE HEALTH™

The Guide to Wellness of Body and Mind

JOSEPH KEON, PH.D.

A Parissound Publication

NOTICE TO THE READER

The author does not directly or indirectly dispense medical advice or prescribe the use of diet as a means of treating disease without prior medical approval. It is not the intent of the author to diagnose or prescribe. The information presented in this book is general and not intended for your specific health problems. If you are seriously ill, please do not make dietary changes without first consulting your medical doctor. It is your constitutional right to make decisions without prior approval from your doctor; however, in such case you are prescribing for yourself, and the publisher and author of this book assume no responsibility. Please consult your physician prior to beginning any exercise program.

Published by:

Parissound Publishing
16 Miller Avenue, Suite 203
Mill Valley, CA 94941, U.S.A.
(415) 383-2884

Library of Congress Catalog Card Number: 95-70987
ISBN 0-9648974-8-2

Whole Health,™ The Whole Health Equation,™ and The Revised American Diet™ are protected trademark names.

Printed in the United States of America

ACKNOWLEDGMENTS

All of the following people, facilities, and organizations played an important role in making *Whole Health* possible.

Peggy Keon; Richard Adamson Lumpkin; Molly Green Lumpkin; Pam Keon, M.S.; Liese A. Keon, M.S.; Susan Keon De Wyngaert, M.D.; Margaret L. Keon; Katherine S. Keon; Evan Frank; Neal Arnove; Claudia Miles; Gynne Stern; Larry Townsend; Mark Binkin; Michael A. Klaper, M.D.; Mark Ferrel; The Cooper Institute for Aerobics Research; Leslie Tilling; Deborah Phelan; Ronald Marquardt, Ph.D.; Keith and Emilie Lord; Michelle Lawrence; Cindy Rockoff; Patricia Waughtal, L.M.S.W.; W. Smith Chandler, M.D., M.S., M.P.H., F.A.C.O.E.M; Elson Haas, M.D.; John Robbins; Paul Yazolino; Barbara Custer, O.M.D.; Mark Lovendale; Betty Musham; Brian Ades; Evette Lowenthal; Derek Barton; Gold's Gym Enterprises, Inc.; Gold's Gym, Marin, CA; World Gym, Marin, CA; Powerhouse Gym, Chatsworth, CA; Fifth Street Fitness, Santa Rosa, CA; Bruce Mossberg; Charlie Carpentar; Sue Porter; Tom Kendrick; Trina Lindsey; Diane Lindsey; Trisha Roloff; Nancy Sundquist; Gina Mansfield; Jennifer Raymond, M.S.; Fabio; Russ Squire; EarthSave Foundation; Diane Scott; Diana Frank; Guillaume Preniaux; Thomas Rhett Kee; Kevin Price; Mary McClure; Marianne Rayburn; Miguel De Lalama, X; Mike Marino; Mike Navone; Nelson Tilling; Paula Crane; Richard Redmond; Paul, John Paul, and Robert at It Talent, Los Angeles, CA; Rick Warner; Sebastian Jackovicks; John Rigelhof; SoYoung Mack; Richard Confalone; Annie Somerville; Garth Twa; Kevin Witt, D.C., C.C.S.P.; Mark Lovendale; Elika Hemphill; Bob DelMonteque; Danielle Shapero, Shahrokh Taleghani, Naghmeh Amir Alikhani, Sue Maunders, Carolyn Keating, Deirdre Gawoski.

Grateful acknowledgment is given to Boehringer Ingelheim International for the right to reprint the blood vessel photo series by Lennart Nilsson on page 40. © Boehringer Ingelheim International GmbH, *The Body Victorious*, Dell Publishing Company.

Grateful acknowledgment is also given to Bantam Doubleday Dell and Annie Somerville for the right to reprint recipes from *Fields of Greens* by Annie Somerville. © 1993 Annie Somerville. Used by permission of Bantam Books, a division of Bantam Doubleday Dell Publishing Group, Inc.

Exercise models: Bill Vetro, Jim Caciola, Daryl Jané, Sheila Joyce, Linda Sobek, Rob McGinnes, Nino Pepicelli, Michelle DeMiranda, Jennifer Warren, Bruce Scottow, Mia Finnegan, Richard Finnegan, Justin D. Dunne, Nicole Bray.

Cover and book design by Danielle Shapero Design, Los Angeles, CA.

Cover photograph: Water-lilies photographed at the home of impressionist Claude Monet, Giverny, France © 1985 Joseph Keon

Unless otherwise indicated, all photography by John Rigelhof.

I am particularly thankful to:

Danielle Shapero for her unswerving support and direction, for gracing this project with her gift for design, and her invaluable friendship.

Sue Porter for being such a great fan, and for being there from the start. I haven't forgotten the horses!

Rich Confalone and Elika Hemphill, my good friends who graciously opened up their home to me on my many trips to Los Angeles during the production process.

Guillaume "Mr. Pull-up" Pruniaux, a great training partner and supreme friend. Thanks for keeping me on course.

Paula Doubleday, for her professionalism, guidance and patience in bringing this project to completion.

For my mother and father.

TABLE OF CONTENTS

BOOK TWO

INTRODUCTION

The doctor of the future will give no medicine, but will interest
his patient in the care of the human frame, in diet, and in
the cause and prevention of disease.
—Thomas Edison

Years ago, I assumed, as many still do, that such ailments as heart disease, cancer, high blood pressure, diabetes, and obesity were conditions one is either born with, genetically predisposed to, or simply unlucky enough to contract. I concurred with the popular belief that osteoporosis, the progressive degeneration of the bones that can lead to crippling hip and spinal fractures, was the consequence of an insufficient intake of calcium and the best antidote would be to double up on the consumption of milk and other dairy products – a prescription I followed, consuming nearly a gallon of the stuff a day. Because my coaches convinced me of the importance of protein for an athlete, I made sure I had plenty of that in my diet as well. I knew the best sources of protein, too: beef, chicken, and eggs.

After becoming certified as a fitness trainer, I was forced to look more closely at the role diet plays in health and fitness. My clients began asking me questions about high-protein diets, low-carbohydrate diets, liquid diets, diets for weight gain, and diets for weight loss. Some of my clients had high blood pressure, others had diabetes. I felt unable to give adequate responses to their questions. This led me to the library to do a bit of research. Little did I know what lay ahead!

What I thought would be a few trips to the public library led to my nearly holding a "post" at the medical school library. A fuse had been lit, and I quickly saw that not only was my understanding of how foods affect human health limited, it was distorted. I felt as though little bombs were going off, one by one, exploding the nutritional myths by which I lived, and by which so many people continue to live today.

As my research continued, I uncovered study upon study that contradicted everything that I had come to "know for certain" about nutrition and its effects on human health. For example, a plethora of scientific studies indicated that the consumption of large quantities of milk and other animal protein is more likely one of the major *causes* of osteoporosis rather than its cure. I discovered that the animal protein I coveted so dearly is highly overrated, widely misunderstood, and consumed far in excess of human needs, and for these reasons, it is a likely contributor to numerous health problems. As I delved into my research, it became clear that not only osteoporosis, but heart disease, stroke, high blood pressure, some forms of cancer, obesity, and even dental disease – diseases that most commonly afflict Americans – are clearly related to the dietary and other lifestyle choices each of us makes.

Countless studies have been conducted worldwide; scientists have submitted their results; the evidence is enormous. Yet I felt I was discovering something that had been buried, and I had a lot of questions. Why was I not aware of this information before? Why are Americans being misled about their health? Was this misinformation deliberate? I became so engrossed by my findings that I decided to return to school and pursue further studies in nutrition.

What I came to understand is that the majority of today's major health problems are not due to chance, but are in fact largely related to lifestyle, and I began to see just how powerful an influence each of us can have over our health. I was alarmed not only at how terribly misinformed the general public is, but also those in the world of healthcare who advise the public about their lifestyle choices.

While it became increasingly clear to me that dietary choices play a powerful role in disease prevention, and that when partnered with exercise the results are even more dramatic, I also came to realize that another aspect was missing from most approaches to achieving and maintaining wellness. To achieve optimum health, one must consider not only the body, but also the mind, and the highly interactional relationship between the two.

As the scope of my understanding of what is necessary to achieve optimal health continued to evolve, I began preparing a manual for my clients and those with whom I was unable to work directly. As with many projects, this one took on a life of its own, and the manual grew into the book you are presently holding. In *Whole Health*, I present to you what I call the Whole Health Equation, the assembly of four components for achieving and maintaining optimal health. The Whole Health Equation addresses nutrition, the muscular system, the cardiovascular system, and the relationship between mind and body. The components are addressed in three distinct yet interdependent sections in this book.

In Book One you will discover the Revised American Diet, and explore how proper nutrition can be one of your most powerful tools in disease prevention. We will examine how the diet followed by the majority of Americans and endorsed by public health organizations (what I refer to as the Standard American Diet [SAD]) is indeed contributing to ill health. You will learn how by making the transition to the Revised American Diet, each of us can dramatically reduce our risk of disease, maintain an abundance of energy, eliminate chronic ailments, and put an end to the miserable yo-yo dieting cycle that traps so many Americans.

In Book Two you will learn about the many benefits of exercising both the muscular and cardiovascular systems. You will learn how to incorporate a lifelong exercise program into your daily schedule, learning the fundamentals of movement and stretching as well as progressive resistance and aerobic exercises. You will gain strength, coordination, and stamina, as well as flexibility, to a degree you may not have thought possible.

In Book Three we will explore the final component of the Whole Health Equation by examining the leading edge in preventive medicine, the relationship between mind and body. In looking at this relationship, you will learn to use such tools as visualization, meditation, relaxation and breathing exercises, goal setting, and time management.

A warning: this is not a "get rich quick" approach to health and fitness. The overnight approaches – the "meal in a can," "breakfast bars," "fat burner pills," rubber-band exercisers, thigh creams, "energy pills," and other such health quackery – have left millions of Americans disillusioned, if not disabled, alongside the road to wellness. Instead, this is a step-by-step approach where we demystify the terms *health* and *fitness*, learn exactly what our minds and bodies need, and discover how best to fulfill those needs in a way that provides lifelong results.

I am very excited about the results Whole Health living is achieving for individuals just like yourself. Those who have made the transition to the Revised American Diet and applied the other components of the Whole Health Equation are healthy, strong, have an abundance of energy, and have left behind forever any former weight problems. Some have reduced or eliminated burdensome medications they thought would always be a part of their lives. More important, they are free of joint pain, headaches, chronic colds, and other bothersome ailments and have significantly reduced their risk of a host of debilitating diseases that plague the American population. The lifelong benefits and protection Whole Health living affords are now available.

If you use it, the information in the following pages can have a tremendous impact on your present and future well-being. It will empower, energize, and heal you, changing your relationship to your body and mind for the rest of your life.

Joseph Keon
Mill Valley, CA
April 18, 1996

CHAPTER ONE

THE WAKE-UP CALL

Maintaining order rather than correcting disorder
is the ultimate principle of wisdom.
– Nei Jing Chinese Medical Text

Whole Health is a wake-up call. First, it will wake us to the realities behind the many myths associated with health and fitness. Second, it will alert us to some very real health problems, not widely known but among the most pressing health issues for Americans today.

In these pages you will discover alarming facts about the health of Americans. For many of you there will be a sense of awakening followed by a desire for change. For others, this book may serve as a confirmation of their current beliefs about personal health or lifestyle changes they have already made.

Change or growth comes about through increased awareness. The more we know, the easier change becomes. This book will provide a greater awareness about the body and mind and what they require to operate in a state of wellness.

Currently, the top ten prescription drugs in America account for more than 160 million of the 1.5 billion prescriptions written annually. Included are such popular drugs as Vasotec®, Lanoxin®, Seldane®, Procardia®, and Zantac®, drugs that treat high blood pressure, heart disease, allergy, angina (chest pain), and ulcers. Perhaps you find this as alarming as I do. Not only are prescriptions dispensed with increasing frequency, but some individuals are taking several prescription drugs simultaneously. In his excellent book *Lifeguide*, David Perlmutter, M.D., reveals that, until recently, the makers of a drug commonly prescribed for angina and hypertension were providing physicians with frequent flyer miles each time they prescribed their drug!

In addition to prescription drugs, Americans consume enormous amounts of over-the-counter remedies – for conditions such as headaches, gas, insomnia, indigestion, and heartburn – that provide only temporary symptomatic relief. I have always felt that if the human body was intended to ingest all these drugs, we would probably find trees with blossoms of Tagament®, Rolaids®, and Alka-Seltzer.®

I'm not saying there is no place for prescription medications. On the contrary, modern medicine has formulated "miracle" drugs that have saved lives and alleviated painful symptoms. The problem is that the bulk of both prescription and over-the-counter drugs are taken for conditions that can largely be prevented in the first place through proper nutrition, exercise, and stress prevention and reduction strategies. Unfortunately, until recently, the emphasis in healthcare has not been on prevention, but instead on treatment and "cure." But like trying to mop up water around an overflowing sink without reaching to turn off the faucet, the task is hopelessly Sisyphean.

Healthcare costs in the United States are quickly moving toward the $1 trillion mark, a cost we simply can no longer afford. While Congress continues to dither about the best strategy to deal with this cost, little has even been mentioned about reducing costs through prevention. Amazing as it sounds, if we were to prevent just 50 percent of the cases of heart disease, stroke, hypertension, cancer, diabetes, osteoporosis, and dental diseases, the United States could be spared over $120 billion in direct and indirect healthcare costs. Can we achieve such a result? The answer is a resounding *yes!* One of the greatest hurdles to such prevention is the lack of information available to the public about how they can prevent these diseases. The public must be presented accurate and useful information that they can use to live more productive lives free of illness and disease.

For too long, people have been duped into believing that these dreaded and debilitating diseases are out of individual control, "part of the life cycle," or worse, that they are diseases of the elderly. When people are able to escape such diseases, we think of them as "lucky." The reality, though, is encouragingly different. Health has little to do with luck. While genetics does play a part, each of us can have a tremendous influence over our health – more than most of us have ever imagined.

Most of us have a litany of reasons to justify our current unhealthy lifestyles. One of the most common is to cite the "good" health of someone we know who lives life in "the fast lane." "You know my buddy Mike smokes two packs of cigarettes a day, drinks whiskey, and eats junk food, and he's in great health." While some people may fool us with a deceptively healthy outward appearance, when you get down to it, they are not healthy at all. Granted, there are people who escape all research and statistics that suggest they should be severely disabled by disease, if not stone cold dead, before their fourth decade. Unfortunately, these people end up being the model to which many of us point when confronted about our own health. Our philosophy becomes "If they can do it and get away with it, so can I!" The unfortunate reality is that those who are "getting away with it" account for a very small part of the population, one that, statistically speaking, is shrinking fast.

Too often disability and disease are accepted by the general public as the inevitable consequence of age. We have an ingrained belief that, as we age, our body will progressively fall apart, our senses will grow faint, our strength will diminish, and our mobility will become restricted. In fact, this is far from the truth. I'm going to paint you a vividly different picture. I cannot count the number of times I have heard statements such as "Well, at my age what do you expect?" or "At my age I shouldn't do anything that physical." In reality, they have it backwards. At any age (given that they have no detrimental physical condition) people can and should be active and exercise regularly.

The truth is, most people die prematurely and often of an illness that could have been prevented. Even more sobering is this: Nobody is at greater risk for premature death than a sedentary individual. It's estimated that only 15 percent of people over the age of 65 are free of major diseases; the remaining 85 percent are suffering from diseases that can largely be prevented through a regular exercise program, relaxation and stress management, and healthy nutrition.

It's ironic that in one of the wealthiest countries in the world our quality of life is so much lower than it could be. I'm not talking about the Lexus, the cellular phone, or the summer house in the country, but our level of wellness – the absence of disease, chronic aches and pains, indigestion, headaches, low energy, numbed senses, lack of mobility, obesity, depression, and other problems. Wellness is a commodity no amount of money can buy. Consider the following:

Every thirty-four seconds a human being dies from cardiovascular disease; that will mean 1 million deaths this year.[1] Over 70 million Americans suffer from one or more forms of vascular disease including coronary heart disease, high blood pressure, rheumatic heart disease, and stroke. If you are an American male, you stand a 50 percent chance of dying of a heart attack – the odds are more favorable in a round of Russian Roulette! In 1994, the cost for treating cardiovascular disease exceeded $28 billion.[2] Cardiovascular disease is the number-one killer in the United States, and its cause is directly related to poor nutrition and lack of exercise. Closely following cardiovascular disease is cancer. While there are a variety of forms of cancer, those that occur most frequently, such as breast, colon, prostate, rectum, and stomach cancer, are all strongly correlated with diet. At the turn of the century, about 4 percent of deaths were cancer related. In 1960, cancer accounted for about 15 percent of all deaths. Experts estimate that at the current rate of increase, unless there is a serious effort toward prevention, 25 percent of deaths will be due to cancer and 40 percent of adults will have some form of cancer by the year 2000. Diabetes, a disease characterized by inadequate production or utilization of insulin, is the most frequent cause of blindness and extremity amputation. In 1992, diabetes costs were estimated to be $92 billion. Osteoporosis is a progressive degeneration of the skeletal system that interferes with the mechanical support function of bone and results in increasingly frequent bone fractures. In advanced cases, a mere sneeze can result in a cracked rib bone. Last year, healthcare costs for this disease far exceeded $10 billion.

Every one of these diseases is strongly associated with poor diet and lack of exercise, meaning that each of us can play a powerful role in their prevention, and in some cases, their reversal. Our health is something that for too long we have left in the hands of others – doctors, pharmacists, and other healthcare professionals – who, more often than not, are in the business of treating diseases *after* they have begun their deleterious course through our bodies. A different way of thinking and acting, outlined in the following pages, is one where we take responsibility for our individual health and seek out every option we have to prevent illness in the first place. We don't need to be doctors or have an extensive education in the dynamics of the human body. We simply need to understand what our bodies require to remain healthy and illness-free and to have the willingness to make a commitment to implement these life-enhancing changes. The fact is, good health – Whole Health – can truly be a pleasure.

CHAPTER TWO

THE WHOLE HEALTH EQUATION ™

In wisdom we look at the whole, in ignorance we look at the parts.
– Plato

WHAT IS WHOLE HEALTH?

Over the years I have come to look at Whole Health as an equation made up of several components. If one or more parts are missing, we fail to get the desired result. Many people are applying only a segment of the total equation, and, consequently, they are unable to achieve optimal health. By the time you finish reading this book, you will know and understand the health equation and how it applies to your pursuit of excellent health.

THE FITNESS FRENZY

In a sporting goods store recently, a salesman tried to convince me that the new athletic shorts he was trying to sell could actually build muscle. "How's that?" I asked him. "You see," he said, "it's in the tightness of the short fabric. As it grips the skin of your thigh and you move, it forces the muscles to contract and works them." I didn't know whether to laugh or not. When I asked the salesman where he learned this, he proudly responded, "The clothing rep."

Folks, let's stop deluding ourselves. Real health and fitness does not come in a pill, diet drink, or protein powder . . . and it certainly does not come from the clothes you wear!

In the 1980s there was an exercise explosion. Motivated by a desire for muscular strength, beauty, endurance, and more recently, control of weight and cholesterol levels, there were more people exercising than ever before. It is estimated that in 1960, 150,000 people exercised regularly. During the '80s estimates approached 36 million. However, as we moved into the '90s, people began to return to their former sedentary ways. In truth, as a population we are largely un-exercised and significantly overweight. Current estimates are that at least 40 percent of the United States population is sedentary, and of the other 60 percent, only about one fifth exercise regularly enough for it to benefit their health.

What does it mean to be healthy? Where does exercise fit in? Do you think that you are in optimal health? Maybe you take long walks. Perhaps you play on a community softball team or get in a couple of games of tennis each week. You may even run or ride a bike. While these are all good fitness activities, no single activity by itself is the key to Whole Health.

WHOLE HEALTH IS COMPRISED OF FOUR COMPONENTS:

1. Proper nutrition
2. Cardiovascular conditioning
3. Muscular conditioning
4. Mental conditioning

Proper nutrition is attained through choosing a variety of wholesome and natural low-fat foods to nourish the body; cardiovascular conditioning is achieved through activities such as running, swimming, and bicycling; muscular conditioning is achieved through stretching, calisthenics, and progressive resistance exercise using free weights and machines; mental conditioning involves using exercises such as meditation, visualization, and stress reduction strategies to move toward a more regular state of mindfulness. Our state of mind may have more impact on wellness than we ever imagined possible.

You may have a terrific physique, but if your heart and lungs are weak and you become winded after climbing a flight of stairs, the equation is incomplete. Furthermore, even with great physical strength and what appears to be a physically fit body, you may be slowly and quietly sabotaging your health through a diet of excessive saturated fats, cholesterol, and other hidden hazards.

CHAPTER THREE

NUTRITION

Your choice of diet can influence your long-term health
prospects more than any other action you might take.
– Former Surgeon General C. Everett Koop

Our eating habits can have a profound impact on our daily lives, as well as on our overall health. Several hundred years ago, it was prophesied that, by the end of the second millennium, medical doctors would no longer be prescribing drugs to their patients but instead would be prescribing diet as a remedy for most maladies. Unfortunately, despite more awareness, that has largely not been the case. In the following chapters you will see how powerfully the foods you choose can affect your health, and how by making certain choices you can protect yourself from the life of accelerated degeneration and disease that afflicts so many Americans.

All of the biochemical processes taking place in our bodies, such as digestion, absorption, transportation, respiration, and metabolism, are highly interdependent and occur in a state of balance or "dynamic equilibrium." When the equilibrium is disrupted, the results can include numerous states of disease. To ensure that this balance is maintained, the body must have an adequate supply of the various nutrients. Excesses or deficiencies of these nutrients are equally disruptive and can have serious consequences on our health.

As we learn more about the human body and its relationship to food and the nutrients it provides, we are finding that what was once considered "healthy" may be considered risky today. For example, in the 1950s a total blood cholesterol level of 350 milligrams per deciliter was considered safe. Today, by conventional wisdom, an individual is considered in risky territory if her total cholesterol level reaches 220. In reality, significant risk exists for an individual at levels below 220. You will learn why later in Chapter Five. Margarine, which came to the rescue in the '80s when butter was indicted as an unhealthy source of saturated fat and cholesterol, has now been identified as problematic because of the trans-fatty acids it contains. Until recently, meat was considered a healthy source of protein and iron – in fact, in this country, meat was once a status symbol. Those who could afford to eat steak were considered "well-off." While this association between meat and wealth is now occurring in developing countries, the story is quite different in the United States. Many Americans seem ready now to face the music – the ample scientific evidence that demonstrates that a meat-centered diet can be detrimental to our health.

After a tremendous amount of research, I have come to agree with Albert Einstein when he said, "Nothing will benefit human health and increase the chances for survival of life on earth as much as the evolution to a vegetarian diet." At this point, some of you may be gasping, "What? Did you say vegetarian?" Yes I did. As author Victoria Moran says, "Eating primarily from the plant kingdom will not change your politics, religion, or any other part of yourself that the label vegetarian doesn't seem to fit." If you stick with me, I believe you'll be enlightened by what you read here, and the idea of eating a vegetarian diet will make perfect sense to you.

Einstein saw very clearly where we have been heading, both in terms of our personal health and the health of the planet. He also knew an effective way to halt this deleterious course. It seems that a significant number of people in the United States are now discovering the same thing. Where once vegetarian cookbooks were obscure, they are currently the fastest-selling cookbooks in national bookstore chains.

Estimates are that there are approximately 11 million vegetarians in the United States today, and hundreds of millions worldwide. The research is conclusive that a vegetarian diet – one that excludes meat, fish, eggs, and dairy products in favor of foods from the plant kingdom – offers not only greater levels of energy, easy weight control, better-looking skin, and a host of other benefits, but more important, significant protection from several chronic, degenerative diseases. The American Dietetic Association agrees that vegetarians have a significantly lower risk of coronary heart disease, hypertension, obesity, diabetes mellitus, osteoporosis, kidney stones, gallstones, and diverticula disease, as well as colon, uterine, and prostate cancer.[3] Recent studies have confirmed that women who consume a vegetarian diet are at lower risk for breast cancer.[4] Even the American Medical Association, considered by many to be extremely conservative in its position, reported as far back as 1961 that 90 percent of incidents of heart disease could be prevented simply by maintaining a vegetarian diet.

There is no question that vegetarians have a higher quality of life. They simply are not burdened with the ailments and illnesses that their non-vegetarian brothers and sisters are commonly afflicted with. So it is no surprise that vegetarians also live longer lives. A massive study conducted by Loma Linda University demonstrated clearly that vegetarians live 10 to 15 years longer than those who eat the "Standard American Diet," that is, the diet of the average American.

Strictly speaking, there are three different degrees of vegetarianism. The closer you move toward complete vegetarianism or veganism (pronounced *vee-gun-ism*), the greater the benefits you'll receive.

Lacto-ovo-vegetarianism: Diet includes dairy products and eggs, along with plant foods.
Lacto-vegetarianism: Diet excludes eggs, but includes dairy products along with plant foods.
Veganism: Veganism is vegetarianism in the purest sense. Diet excludes all meats, poultry, fish, eggs, and dairy products – any food derived from the animal kingdom. Vegans enjoy the greatest health benefits.

A vegetarian diet is:

- High in complex carbohydrates
- High in fiber
- Rich in vitamins and minerals
- Rich in antioxidants and phytochemicals

- Low in fat, particularly the saturated variety
- Low in sodium
- Low in (or without) cholesterol

Seventh-Day Adventists are a group that has been closely studied and who have become a model of the benefits of the vegetarian diet. One study reveals that Seventh-Day Adventists between the ages of 35 and 64 enjoy a 72 percent reduction in risk of mortality from coronary heart disease, the number-one killer in America.

Not only is the vegetarian at lower risk for the health problems listed above, but since a vegetarian diet is naturally low in fat, it is extremely rare to find a vegetarian who is overweight. We will look more closely at this topic in Chapter Eight.

The vegetarian lifestyle is becoming increasingly popular in the United States and has been enjoyed for thousands of years by millions of people. In fact, some of the greatest and most influential figures in history have been vegetarians. See if you recognize some of them:[5]

Dustin Hoffman	Cesar Chavez	Susan B. Anthony
Charles Darwin	Albert Schweitzer	Laura Huxley
Leo Tolstoy	Pythagoras	Paul McCartney
Plato	George Bernard Shaw	Socrates
Vincent van Gogh	Cicily Tyson	Henry David Thoreau
Leonardo da Vinci	Ralph Waldo Emerson	Mahatma Gandhi
Albert Einstein	Sting	Benjamin Franklin

You may be saying to yourself, "But I'm an athlete. There's no way I can build muscle and strength, let alone perform well as a vegetarian." You may feel differently when you learn of these vegetarian athletes:

Dave Scott: *Six-time winner of the Ironman Triathlon*

Sixto Linares: *World record holder, 24-hour Triathlon*

Paavo Nurmi: *World record distance runner, nine Olympic medals*

Henry Aaron: *Major League Baseball champion*

Robert Parish: *Boston Celtics, starting center*
Stan Price: *World record-bench press*
Andreas Cahling: *"Mr. International" title holder, body building*
Roy Hilligan: *"Mr. America" title holder, body building*
Bill Pearl: *"Mr. America," "Mr. Universe" title holder, body building*
Carl Lewis: *Olympic track champion*

CHAPTER FOUR

WHAT'S WRONG WITH THE STANDARD AMERICAN DIET?

We, as scientists, can no longer take the attitude that the public cannot benefit from information they are not ready for.
– T. Colin Campbell, Ph.D.

Due to misinformation, the average American follows by default a diet I call the Standard American Diet. The acronym for the Standard American Diet (SAD) speaks for itself. The average person today knows very little about the foods he or she eats. Consequently, many of us make food choices based on convenience, price, availability, perhaps even packaging. In doing so, we are placing a great deal of unwarranted trust in those food producers and organizations that are often merely looking to make a profit.

Unfortunately, such unconscious dietary habits put many people into a state of malnutrition. Most people probably associate this term with the heartrending pictures of third-world children with distended bellies. The fact is, malnutrition means not only a lack of vital nutrients but an excess and imbalance of them as well, and the potential consequences are numerous: most seriously, heart disease, cancer, high blood pressure, diabetes, dental complications, and gastrointestinal disorders. The great news is that in most cases, through healthy eating habits, each of us can prevent or positively affect these disorders!

If asked whether they consume a nutritious diet, most people would probably say they do. "Of course, I do have a little ice cream every now and then," they might confide, adding, "but it's that healthy kind; you know, the gourmet stuff."

Here's the truth. The Standard American Diet contains: up to 42 percent of its calories as fat, 130 pounds of sugar a year, four times the body's daily protein requirement (two-thirds of which comes from animal sources high in fat and cholesterol), and about 500 percent of the body's sodium requirement. The result is a nutritional disaster. The United States has one of the highest rates in the world for coronary heart disease, heart attack, stroke, cancer, high blood pressure, diabetes, obesity, osteoporosis, and tooth decay – all nutrition-related diseases.

If we were to isolate the single factor most responsible for diet-related disease, without question it would be the consumption of excess fat and cholesterol. As the consumption of fat and cholesterol-rich animal products has increased, it has displaced the ingestion of plant foods naturally rich in the health-giving components we know as vitamins, minerals, phytochemicals, and fiber. Yet things weren't always this way – they've changed a great deal since the turn of the century.

HOW THINGS HAVE CHANGED

At the beginning of the century, the average diet contained about 50 percent more grain food than it does today, while plant foods accounted for about half the total protein consumed. Today, animal foods supply about two-thirds of the total protein consumed. As the consumption of grain products, vegetables, legumes, and nuts has dropped, the consumption of meat, poultry, and soft drinks has risen markedly. What's worse, the level of fat in the food supply has increased 30 percent. Just 30 years ago, the average person consumed about 30 pounds more fresh fruit and 20 pounds more fresh vegetables a year than they do today. Currently it's estimated that, in one year, the United States consumes the contents of 90 million jars and cans and 40 million pounds of frozen and packaged foods – foods that are nutritionally inferior to the fresh, whole foods they have come to displace.

We rely on the purveyors of foods to tell us what is nutritious, but due to a conflict of interest, this is not always smart. For instance, the Meat Board is probably not the best source for information about human protein needs, yet it, along with the American Dairy Council, provides free nutrition education materials to schools and spends hundreds of millions of dollars on advertisements to convince people to depend on its products. Consequently, many of us have grown up with an approach to nutrition strongly influenced by these biases. No wonder so many people make poor choices when it comes to what they eat.

A recent study clearly illustrates the confusion over nutrition. This study is particularly alarming because it involves those who may play a crucial role in the development of eating habits in adolescents. In the study, high school and college physical education teachers and coaches were given a questionnaire to determine their nutritional knowledge. Over one-third of those questioned believed that protein is the primary source of muscular energy.[6] In truth, carbohydrates are the primary source of energy, followed by fats. Protein actually contributes the least to energy needs as it is reserved for the maintenance of tissues. Most of the instructors who answered this survey believed that they had a strong influence on their students' eating habits. This is truly unfortunate. In a later section, we'll look at how the protein myth has contributed to several health problems.

CURRENT DIETARY RECOMMENDATIONS AND WHY THEY ARE FAILING

In order to provide some dietary guidance for Americans, the Recommended Dietary Allowances (RDA) were established and have been continually revised by the Food and Nutrition Board of the National Academy of Sciences, National Research Council, over the last 60 years.

While one might expect that refinement over the years has led to significant improvement in our understanding of nutrition and thus our health, such is not the case. Current recommendations contain far too many calories from animal-source foods, which are low in important fiber, and naturally high in saturated fat and cholesterol – two factors that influence the progression of human disease. Nutrient proportion recommendations have also been made in terms of the percentage of calories one should consume daily from each of the primary nutrient groups: proteins, fats, and carbohydrates. Although the latest figures are endorsed by numerous public health organizations, they still miss the mark.

Recommended intakes of the dietary nutrients have been consistently high, as each nutrient recommendation has included a "margin of safety." As an example, let's look at protein. The World Health Organization of the United Nations recommends that protein intake be 4.5 percent of total calories consumed; the Food and Nutrition Board of the U.S. Department of Agriculture suggests 6 percent of total calories. At the high end, the National Research Council suggests 8 percent of total calories consumed should be in the form of protein. However, Americans are consistently being told by public health organizations that they should consume 15 percent of their calories as protein.

Last year I attended a conference at which a researcher from one of the country's most respected health institutions was speaking. During the presentation, he cited numerous studies showing the relationship between a high-fat diet and the onset of many of the degenerative diseases I have mentioned. At the conclusion of his presentation, he recommended that individuals strive to keep their fat intake to 30 percent of their total calories. (This, incidentally, is the same recommendation that the Senate Select Committee on Nutrition and most public health organizations in America stand by.) Later I approached him with a concern. I explained that, based on the significant and extensive data he had just presented, it seemed that we should actually be advising people to further decrease their fat intake – perhaps closer to 15 percent of their daily calories. Without hesitation, he agreed. He then commented on the fact that the National Academy of Sciences Committee on Diet, Nutrition and Cancer had chosen the level purely for practicality, not because there was research suggesting the figure was appropriate. In fact, *no studies exist that support a 30 percent intake of fat.* The logic in designating this figure was based on the fact that the average American consumes around 40 percent of his or her calories as fat, and therefore, a 10 percent reduction is a "reasonable expectation" – a change that is believed to be achievable. Asking people to reduce their fat intake further, he explained, was seen as too demanding and, therefore, likely to be unsuccessful.

I walked away from that conference a bit bewildered. Later I would discover that in the executive summary of the National Academy's 1982 report it was stated,

"The scientific data do not provide a strong basis for establishing fat intake at precisely 30 percent of total calories. Indeed, the data could be used to justify an even greater reduction."[7] Why, then, are we guiding people toward a recommended fat intake that is higher than what we know is healthy?

A study was conducted by noted cardiologist Dr. Dean Ornish and his colleagues in which participants who were already experiencing repercussions of a high-fat diet (namely, atherosclerosis or "hardening of the arteries") were placed on a diet in which they consumed 30 percent of their calories as fat. The result was that not only did the subjects not show signs of recovery from this change, but their condition continued to worsen. Further, an important Harvard University study reported in the *New England Journal of Medicine* that a diet consisting of 30 percent of calories as fat offered no measurable reduction in the risk of cancer.[8]

Recommendations for a daily cholesterol intake of 300 mg have just as little foundation to support them. Again, this is simply an arbitrary number that has been chosen to guide Americans. You will soon see that it is a dangerous recommendation.

CHAPTER FIVE

DISEASES AND DIET

Clearly, if disease is manmade, it can also be man-prevented.
– Dr. Ernst Wunder

Prior to 1950, the infectious diseases pneumonia, influenza, and tuberculosis were the diseases one was most concerned about. At that time, these were the major causes of untimely death. Today things are very different. Although there has been a resurgence of such diseases as tuberculosis, and we face a tremendous threat from AIDS, no longer are infectious diseases the major threat to life – in fact, they currently account for about 3 percent of deaths.[9] Today the major causes of death are chronic degenerative diseases such as heart disease, cancer, and diabetes. While in 1900 chronic diseases accounted for 14 percent of all deaths, 75 percent of deaths in the United States today can be attributed to a chronic disease; that is, diseases that are strongly related to diet and lifestyle and therefore can be prevented. Let's examine a few of the most prevalent diseases to see how they are perpetuated.

CANCER

The American Cancer Society reports that cancer takes a life every 60 seconds in the United States. Several types of cancer have been linked to diet, specifically dietary fat, including cancer of the breast, prostate, uterus, ovaries, rectum, and colon. The National Cancer Institute estimates this diet-cancer relationship to account for 35 percent of all cancers; some researchers place that figure closer to 60 percent.

Cancer occurs when damaged cells proliferate in an unregulated manner in the body. The damage occurs to the DNA, which is found in the nucleus of every cell. DNA can be thought of as the "brain" of the cell, directing it in its function.

There are numerous agents capable of causing cellular damage – some of the most common include toxic chemicals and radiation. Normally, both tumor suppressor genes and specialized cells in our immune system are on patrol for cancerous cells. When they locate them, these cancerous cells are disposed of and the threat eliminated. However, for various reasons, the efficiency of both of these kinds of patrollers can be compromised, and a damaged cell can be allowed to proliferate, one cell becoming two, two becoming four, and so on. This can occur in any tissue of the body, most commonly the lungs, breasts, stomach, colon, prostate, and uterus. In time, the proliferation of cancerous cells can spread to other damage-free cells in the body, eventually creating total cellular havoc. With modern medicine, the presence of cancer is not necessarily a death warrant; however, in many cases the disease is not discovered until it reaches a point where treatment has little effect.

BREAST CANCER

The leading cause of premature death for women in the United States is now breast cancer. Since 1965, there has been a 50 percent increase in breast cancer, with the disease now striking one in eight women. This year, 185,000 women will be diagnosed as having breast cancer.[10]

Breast cancer is a multifactorial disease. Aside from genetic background, early menarche, late pregnancy (or no pregnancy), height and weight, X rays (specifically mammograms), pesticides, toxic chemicals, estrogen replacement therapy (ERT), birth control pills, alcohol, and poor diet are known risk factors.

The reality is that mainstream medicine has been quite vocal in regard to early breast cancer detection. The voice of prevention, however, has been barely audible. Contrary to what most women have been lead to believe, the truth is that with the right information, they can do much to prevent this disease.

Like prostate, uterine, and ovarian cancer, breast cancer is a hormonally regulated cancer. Considerable evidence indicates that a high-fat diet causes an elevation in the level of the hormone estrogen in women. As the level of estrogen goes up, so does the likelihood of breast cancer. The association between fat intake and breast cancer is particularly strong with saturated fat – the type found in animal products.[11] Research findings presented at the United States-Japan Cooperative Cancer Research Conference indicate that a woman who consumes meat on a daily basis is three-and-a-half times more likely to develop breast cancer than a woman who consumes meat less than once a week.[12] When we graph the rates for breast cancer throughout the world, it becomes clear that in areas where fat consumption is highest (particularly saturated animal fats), there are correspondingly higher rates for breast cancer.

When women are placed on moderate-fat diets, something wonderful happens to their estrogen levels: they drop. With this drop comes a reduction in cancer risk. While the presence of estrogen is critical to the health of both men and women, the key is keeping the natural estrogen levels in balance. To assist in this task, the body contains molecules known as sex hormone binding globulins (SHBG). Also known as *carrier molecules*, SHBG can be thought of as a coach who maintains the team member balance on the playing field. When estrogen is needed, it supplies it. When estrogen is not needed, SHBG takes estrogen "out of the game." Clearly, those who consume diets rich in animal fat have lower levels of SHBG available. Conversely, those who consume a vegetarian diet are found to have higher levels of the carrier molecules. In a high-fat diet estrogen levels are elevated, which encourages tumor growth, and the subsequent reduction of carrier molecules that normally would be helping to maintain an estrogen balance.

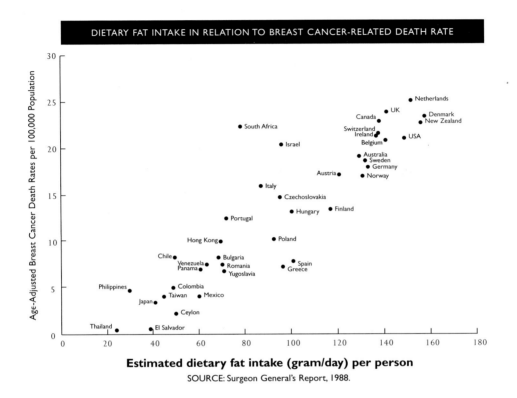

DIETARY FAT INTAKE IN RELATION TO BREAST CANCER-RELATED DEATH RATE

Estimated dietary fat intake (gram/day) per person

SOURCE: Surgeon General's Report, 1988.

While dietary fat clearly has a powerful influence on the development of breast cancer, it is not the only risk factor. Some researchers have suggested that the estrogenic feeds given to farm animals that end up in meat may also contribute to the problem.[13] Currently, it is estimated that 90 percent of chickens, 80 percent of veal calves and hogs, and more than half of all beef cattle are given hormones either as implants or by way of hormone-supplemented feed. Roy Hertz, a hormonal cancer specialist and former Director of Endocrinology of the National Cancer Institute, explains that there are great "carcinogenic risks of estrogenic feeds, particularly for hormonally sensitive tissues such as breast tissue, because they could increase normal body hormonal levels and disturb delicately poised hormonal balances."

ESTROGEN REPLACEMENT THERAPY (ERT)

Many post-menopausal women are advised to begin estrogen therapy to assist in the prevention of osteoporosis and heart disease. While the risks and benefits have been debated for years, a recent Harvard Medical School study led by Graham Colditz demonstrated that such therapy (even when estrogen and progestin are administered together [hormone replacement therapy]) may actually increase the risk of breast cancer by one third or more.[14] While some experts feel more studies are necessary, one thing remains clear: women can significantly lower their risk of heart disease and osteoporosis simply by adopting the lifestyle changes presented in this book.

THE RADIATION CONNECTION

Forty years ago, X-ray machines emitted considerably larger doses of radiation than today's equipment. Today, the sophisticated machinery used emits only a fraction of past levels. However, this does not mean that X rays are harmless. Mammograms (breast X rays) do emit radiation, which is a risk factor for breast cancer. The question is, do the risks outweigh the benefits? Many will argue they do. Others will cite the fact that mammograms are not always accurate, even failing to detect tumors in some cases. While the controversy continues, one thing is certain. Mammograms are one way of *detecting* breast cancer, but they do nothing to *prevent* the disease, and may even be a contributing factor to it.

THE CHEMICAL CONNECTION

We have evolved into a chemical culture, dousing, spraying, and rubbing chemicals on everything around us from our kitchen countertops and automobile tires to the hair on our heads. Hundreds of thousands of chemicals, many of which are suspected carcinogens, are available to the average consumer for daily use. Dr. Devra Lee Davis, Disease Prevention Advisor to the U.S. Department of Health and Human Services, says that many of these chemicals may mimic the effects of estrogen or cause the body to manufacture a "bad" form of estrogen. Most recently indicted are the chemical hair dyes that millions of people use monthly to maintain a particular hair color. Numerous drugs, including antibiotics and others used to treat farm animals, have also been cited as risk factors for cancer, along with the plethora of chemicals used by farmers to protect crops. The number of pesticides, fungicides, and herbicides in use is in the hundreds, and overall usage has increased 3,300 percent since 1945.[15] Nearly 70 percent of these chemicals have been declared carcinogens by the FDA. In a study they conducted, 48 percent of the most popular fruits and vegetables were found to contain chemical pesticide residues.[16] In a recent study of the relationship between breast cancer and pesticides, H. Leon Bradlow, biochemist with the Strang Cancer Prevention Center, Cornell University Medical School, confirmed that the effect of pesticides on the production of "bad" estrogen "was 3-4 times as great as that of a known human carcinogen that was used as a comparison." We will look more closely at the pesticide risk and how to protect yourself from it in Chapter Ten.

Many chemicals, whether inhaled as fumes from a household cleaner, eaten in our foods, or absorbed through our skin, have been found to concentrate themselves in the fatty tissues of the body, and the breast is one prime area. Since a mother's body utilizes its fat reservoirs in producing breast milk, one can learn about body chemical stores in women by sampling their breast milk. Back in 1976, when the chemical DDT was still in rampant use, a study conducted by the Environmental Protection Agency (EPA) found "significant concentrations" in over 99 percent of mothers' milk tested.[17] A similar study in 1981 found high levels of another chemical called polychlorinated biphenyls (PCBs) in all of the one thousand mothers tested.[18]

The good news is this: Vegetarian mothers consistently have lower levels of chemical residues. As for pesticide residues, one study found the milk of vegetarian mothers to contain only 8 percent of the national average.[19] Clearly, the elimination of animal products from the diet will significantly reduce the levels of chemicals being ingested. However, chemical residues found on fruits and vegetables must also be considered. Later we will look at strategies for avoiding these chemicals entirely. In Chapter Nineteen we will look at the relationship between breast cancer and exercise.

PROSTATE CANCER

Like breast cancer, prostate cancer is on the rise, with statistics for the disease now showing rates nearly as high as those for breast cancer. While prostate cancer rates were increasing 8 percent a year between 1986 and 1989, the annual rate of increase doubled in 1990. About one in ten men is being stricken with this disease. While breast cancer appears to now affect even younger women, prostate cancer mostly strikes men over 50 years of age.

The prostate gland has one job to do and that is to produce semen, the vehicle in which sperm cells travel. Like breast cancer, prostate cancer is affected by hormone levels. While men's bodies do contain the female hormone estrogen, the male hormone testosterone also plays a significant role in this disease. As indicated earlier, all hormone levels are altered by diet, specifically by the intake of fat.

A joint study conducted by scientists from Harvard University and the Mayo Clinic has indicated a strong correlation between the consumption of red meat and prostate cancer in men. The study, which included 47,000 men, found that those who consume red meat five or more times per week increased their chance of developing prostate cancer by 2.5 times.[20] While this is an important finding, it is essential to point out that the fat we are concerned with is not limited to that found in meat, but includes the fat in all animal products, including poultry, eggs, milk, cream, butter, and cheese.

So where are cases of prostate cancer the lowest? By now, you may have guessed – in the countries with the lowest consumption of animal fat, and a high intake of dietary fiber. In rural areas of China, for example, rates of prostate cancer are 25 times lower than those in the United States.[21]

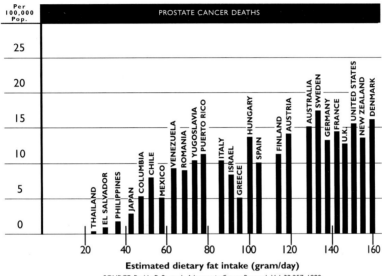

SOURCE: Reddy, B. S., et al., *Advances in Cancer Research*, Vol. 32:257, 1980

We can see how elevated levels of dietary fat work to alter hormone levels within the body. In addition, there is another external source that may be influencing hormone levels: beef.

As previously mentioned, beef cattle are routinely treated with hormones, both natural and artificial. These include testosterone, progesterone, and estradiol, as well as a popular synthetic known as Zeranol.® Cattle breeders use such drugs to produce a larger animal in a shorter period of time, to bring cows into heat for breeding, and to increase milk yields. The hormones are administered by injection, implantation, and in animal feed.[22] Consumers are largely kept in the dark because there are no warning labels required on meat, fish, and poultry informing them of the various chemicals used in processing. Because the effects of consuming tainted meats are largely cumulative and delayed, it may take years before such effects reveal themselves.

COLON CANCER

When the rates of colon cancer are graphed on an international basis, we find yet again that those areas with the highest consumption of fat, particularly animal fat, have the highest number of cases of the disease. Colon cancer is different from breast and prostate cancer in that it is not hormone-regulated.

Of all of the animal-based foods that contribute to cancer, it appears that meat has the most potent role in the development of colon cancer. With no dietary fiber and a great deal of fat, meat is digested more slowly than high-fiber carbohydrate foods like whole grains. It also moves through the digestive tract at a snail's pace in a process called transit time. Normally when the body works to absorb fat, the gallbladder releases bile acids into the intestine, which make the fat assimilable. However, something happens when the fat of meat sits in the intestinal tract too long. A bacteria begins to form and interact with the bile acids, forming carcinogenic products known as secondary bile acids.

A study in the *New England Journal of Medicine* found that women who consume red meat at least once a day double their risk of developing colon cancer. Yet meat is not the only culprit. Numerous studies confirm that the saturated fat found in eggs, fish, poultry, milk, cheese, cream, and butter is also responsible. Again, if we look at China as a model (where animal fat intake is one of the lowest in the world), we see that colon cancer rates are four times lower than in the United States.[23]

Numerous migrational studies have looked at cancer rates for those persons who move to the United States and adopt the "Western diet." One particular study looked at the incidence of colon cancer for Puerto Ricans who have migrated to the United States. In the period between 1958 and 1979, colon cancer mortality rates increased 212 percent in Puerto Rican men and 54 percent in Puerto Rican women who lived in New York City, while rates for those residing in Puerto Rico showed only a slight increase.[24]

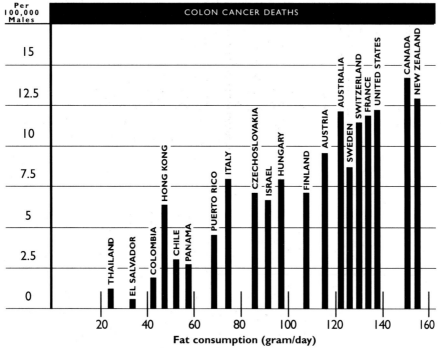

SOURCE: Carroll, K., *Cancer Research*, vol. 35, 1975; Reddy, B. S., et al., *Advances in Cancer Research*, vol. 32:237, 1980

For years researchers have compared the prevalence of nutrition-related disease in the United States, a country that consumes one-third of the world's meat supply, with Asian nations, where the consumption of meat and other animal products (and thus fat) has traditionally been very low. Next to Thailand, China has maintained some of the lowest rates of breast, colon, and prostate cancer, as well as heart disease, in the world. However, the tide is now turning. The reason why is that

Asia is quickly becoming "Americanized" by fast-food chains, convenience foods, and a growing importation of American beef — all sources of saturated fat, cholesterol and chemical residues. As the scientific community has expected, these countries are now experiencing a significant increase in the above diseases.

CORONARY HEART DISEASE

46 percent of all American men at age twenty-two already have the beginnings of coronary heart disease.
– Dr. Tazewell Banks, General Hospital, Washington, D.C.

Coronary heart disease is responsible for 80 percent of all cardiac-related deaths, and in nearly 40 percent of all cases, the first "symptom" of the disease is death. Even though there has been a 40 percent drop in the number of cases since 1968, coronary heart disease remains the number-one killer in America, taking more lives than all forms of cancer combined.[25]

Coronary Heart Disease (CHD) is called "the silent killer" because it can progress to advanced stages without any indication of its presence. CHD is brought about by atherosclerosis (*athero* meaning "paste" and *sclerosis* meaning "thickening" or "hardening"), or what is more commonly referred to as "hardening of the arteries," a process in which the coronary arteries (arteries that supply blood to the heart) undergo a gradual narrowing, reducing the blood supply to the heart. This narrowing of the arterial channel is brought about by a progressive buildup of a plaque composed of cholesterol, fat, damaged cells, and other debris, and is primarily the result of a diet high in saturated fat and cholesterol. While more serious stages of the disease may be detected by increased blood pressure or chest pain (pectoris angina), it is possible for the disease to progress significantly while the host remains symptom-free.

When the arteries to the heart become constricted, there is increased resistance to blood flow, and the heart must work harder to pump blood through the narrowed passage. In unchecked cases, this arterial plaque may become so great that one or

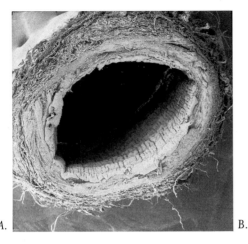

A.

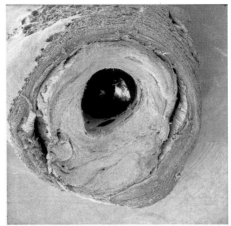

B.

Atherosclerosis. Scanning electron micrographs of cross sections of blood vessels.

A. Healthy vein. Notice the different muscle layers (*top left*).

B. Plaque deposits have reduced space inside the blood vessel, the lumen, by three quarters (*top right*).

C. Blood flow is no longer possible in this totally blocked blood vessel (*bottom right*).

C.

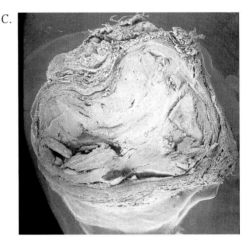

more arteries feeding the heart can become entirely blocked, preventing blood from reaching the heart. Since blood is carrying oxygen to the heart, a complete blockage will result in a myocardial infarction, or what is more commonly known as a heart attack. While not all heart attacks are fatal, they are all serious, since the portion of the heart deprived of blood supply dies.

This same narrowing process can occur in the arteries of the brain. Blockage of these arteries will result in the death of a portion of the brain, a condition known as a stroke. Stroke is the third leading cause of death in the United States and results in serious disability in those who survive.

Every 34 seconds an American dies of a heart attack, and the average American man carries a 50 percent risk of death from this occurrence.[26] That risk drops to 15 percent if he excludes meat entirely from his diet, while a man who consumes no meat, dairy products, or eggs reduces his risk to only 4 percent.[27]

Don't be fooled, as some people have, into thinking CHD is "a disease of the elderly." CHD starts its deleterious course as early as the first decade of life, striking men and women of all ages. In addition to diet, several risk factors may contribute to the onset of CHD.

(1) *Gender:* Men have a higher risk of developing CHD than women, who seem to be better protected from CHD by their sex hormones. At the onset of menopause, however, their risk level begins to climb, and usually will equal that of a similar-aged man.

(2) *Age:* Age is a factor for both men and women. For men 35-65 years of age, the risk increases twofold with each decade. For women 45-65, the risk increases threefold with each decade.

(3) *Heredity:* Those who have a history of cardiovascular disease in their family run a greater risk of developing the disease themselves.

(4) *Cigarette smoking:* Although smoking is more often associated with lung cancer, it also significantly influences the onset of CHD. Smokers more than double their chance of developing CHD. According to the American Heart Association, in 1988, 200,000 people died from cardiovascular disease caused by smoking. Additionally, it was estimated that 37,000 non-smokers died from cardiovascular disease due to

secondhand smoke in their environment.[28] In addition, research has shown that those who smoke and suffer a heart attack are more likely to die from the event than those who don't smoke.

(5) *High blood pressure:* Individuals who have high blood pressure (hypertension) force their heart to work overtime to deliver blood throughout the body. High blood pressure both weakens and enlarges the heart over time.

(6) *Obesity:* Those who are significantly overweight are at greater risk of developing CHD. Survival rates for obese people with CHD are 50 percent lower than for those with a "desirable" body weight. The primary reason is that the excess weight places great strain on the heart, and those who are overweight usually have both high blood cholesterol and high blood pressure as well. Further, those who are significantly overweight run a higher risk of developing diabetes, a risk factor itself.

(7) *Diabetes mellitus:* Those with diabetes carry a twofold risk of developing CHD. Also, because a diabetic experiences abnormal glucose tolerance, their chance of surviving CHD is lower than for a non-diabetic.

The more factors affecting a person, the greater the risk for disease. For instance, a man with high blood pressure doubles his risk for developing CHD. If that same man smoked, his risk would quadruple. If the man were also obese, his risk would be another two to eight times higher than the person without these risks.

In severe cases, medical doctors have two choices for treating atherosclerosis. First, they can perform a procedure known as an angioplasty, where a balloon-tipped catheter is inserted into the artery and then inflated, causing the narrowed portion of the artery to widen. A second option is to take a portion of plaque-free artery from elsewhere in the body and bypass the plaque-narrowed portion of the artery in a process known as coronary artery bypass surgery. I'm sure you would agree that neither approach sounds like much fun. Over 400,000 bypass surgeries are performed annually, and of the patients, about 70 percent are men.[29] Unfortunately, within five years of bypass surgery, unless the patient makes a radical change in his or her lifestyle, the majority of "repaired" arteries become clogged again. The same goes for angioplasty.

Fortunately, you can easily prevent this degenerative process from occurring in the first place. Even if you are already experiencing the effects of atherosclerosis, you may be relieved to know that programs applying a similar diet to the one proposed in this book, in conjunction with other lifestyle changes, have successfully caused a reversal in advanced cases of atherosclerosis. The most well-known is the Lifestyle Heart Trial led by Dr. Dean Ornish at the Preventive Medicine Research Institute.

CHOLESTEROL

Of all the factors we have considered, the most influential and direct link to this disease seems to be dietary. Strong evidence indicates that the higher one's blood cholesterol level, the higher the chance of developing atherosclerotic lesions. Cholesterol levels are increased by dietary fat (specifically the saturated variety) and by cholesterol, which is found only in animal products. Conversely, blood cholesterol levels decrease when saturated fat and cholesterol intake is reduced.

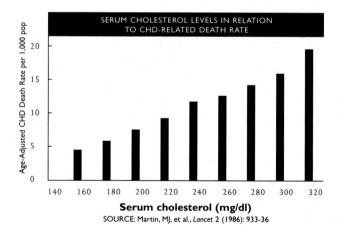

SOURCE: Martin, MJ, et al., *Lancet* 2 (1986): 933-36

A soft waxy material, cholesterol plays a key role in the formation of cell walls, nerve insulation, and the production of steroid hormones and bile acids. The liver is perfectly capable of manufacturing enough cholesterol for the body's needs and does not require excess cholesterol from animal foods. Normally, a "feedback regulator" instructs the liver to reduce production as dietary cholesterol increases. However, the liver is limited in this capacity. The rate at which arterial plaque forms can depend largely on an individual's ability to metabolize dietary fat and cholesterol.

When we consume fats in our diet, they are eventually distributed throughout the body by way of the blood. However, because blood is largely composed of water, and fats and water don't mix, the fats must be repackaged for transportation. The fats are therefore combined into a particle along with two traveling companions, protein and cholesterol. In their repackaged form, the fats are now called lipoproteins (lipo meaning "fat"), and include VLDL, LDL, and HDL. The number and balance of these lipoproteins are different in each body and may be influenced by heredity, diet, and exercise. The problem is that one of these lipoproteins (LDL) is particularly undesirable in large quantities.

VLDL (very low-density lipoproteins) are the largest of the three lipoproteins and are manufactured primarily in the liver. They contain a large amount of triglyceride (fat). As VLDL particles travel throughout the bloodstream, their fat payload is gradually distributed to cells to be used as energy. What remains is a base of cholesterol and protein forming the **LDL (low-density lipoproteins)** particles. Here is where the problem begins. The longer the LDL particles remain in circulation, the greater the chance that they will deposit their cholesterol onto the walls of the arteries, adding to whatever plaque already exists. The greater the deposits, the greater the plaque, and consequently, the narrower the artery becomes. Hence, LDL has earned the name "bad cholesterol."

How long the LDL particles will remain circulating in the blood is primarily determined by a specialized protein called an LDL receptor. Located on the surface of some cells and acting like magnets, LDL receptors bind with the circulating LDL particles and remove them from the bloodstream. Once inside the cell, the cholesterol is broken down. Again, heredity determines the number of LDL receptors we have,

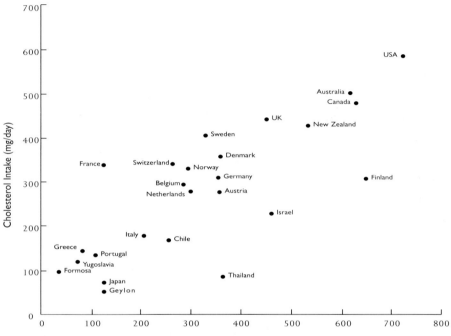

DIETARY CHOLESTEROL INTAKE IN RELATION TO CHD-DEATH RATE

CHD-related death rate per 100,000 male pop. (Age 55-59)
SOURCE: Connor, W. *Preventive Medicine* 1 (1972): 48-83.

and in some individuals, such as those with familial hypercholesterolemia, there is a significant deficiency of LDL receptors.

Hypercholesterolemia occurs when the body is unable to manufacture the LDL receptor proteins sufficiently. Consequently, levels of LDL cholesterol in the blood become critical, resulting in advanced atherosclerosis and sometimes even childhood death.

HDL (high-density lipoproteins), the smallest of the three, are really the heroes in this process. Made of about 50 percent protein, they act like a street cleaner, sweeping through the bloodstream and removing LDL particles and cholesterol, and returning them to the liver where they are broken down into bile acids and eventually excreted. Every time a cell dies and degenerates, it releases its cholesterol payload. HDL then picks up that payload and gets rid of it. So HDL effectively lowers the risk of atherosclerosis. Interestingly, women tend to have measurably higher levels of HDL ("good cholesterol") than men. This is why, for a period in their lives, women remain at much lower risk for heart disease than men. However, following menopause, women begin to catch up.

So how do we prevent CHD? Numerous studies have confirmed that in those societies where dietary fat is kept to a minimum, CHD is relatively rare. For instance in China, where the level of fat intake has traditionally been very low (about 12 percent of total calories come from fat and only 3 percent of total fat is of the saturated variety), CHD rates have been among the lowest in the world. This type of diet can be contrasted with the Standard American Diet, which gets as much as 42 percent of its total calories from fat, about 15-20 percent coming from the saturated variety. The Finnish population consumes even greater quantities of saturated fat than we do in the United States, and their rate of coronary heart disease exceeds that of the United States. There have been no reports of populations where saturated fat and cholesterol levels were high and CHD was not prevalent.

Similar to the change in cancer risk noted earlier, studies show that those who migrate to the United States from areas with low-fat and low-cholesterol diets often adopt the "Western diet" and, consequently, develop the high-risk profile for CHD.

If you have no idea what your current blood cholesterol level is, you should see your physician and have it accurately measured. This is considered to be the most effective way of predicting heart attack risk. Total cholesterol value is determined by the sum of the three lipoproteins: VLDL, LDL, and HDL. The most recent total cholesterol values were established at the National Consensus Conference on Cholesterol in 1985 and are as follows:

AGE	MILLIGRAMS
20	<150 mg/dl
20-29	<180 mg/dl
>30	<200 mg/dl

Current estimates are that 94 million American adults have cholesterol levels above 200 mg/dl, and 37 million have levels that exceed 240 mg/dl.[30]

Some people are misled by the recommended cholesterol levels. They believe that they simply need to bring their cholesterol to what is called an "acceptable range," currently about 200 mg/dl. This is not an acceptable cholesterol level, but was chosen because experts saw it as "attainable." The sad news is that people with cholesterol levels of 200, 190, or even 185 are still having heart attacks.

TOTAL CHOLESTEROL	
AVERAGE HEART ATTACK VICTIM	244 mg/dl
AVERAGE AMERICAN ADULT	205 mg/dl
AVERAGE VEGETARIAN	150 mg/dl

While bringing your cholesterol level down to 180 or even 170 is certainly a move in the right direction, the diet I prescribe in this book, when combined with the other components of the Whole Health Equation, will enable you to bring your cholesterol level even lower – closer to the level it might have been when you were a teenager – about 150 mg/dl. Guess what happens to people who live in the "150 neighborhood"? They don't have heart attacks. One of the most important studies on heart disease is the famous Framingham Heart Study, which has been in progress for over 40 years. Over the years this study has been conducted, not one person with a cholesterol level of 150 or less has experienced a heart attack.

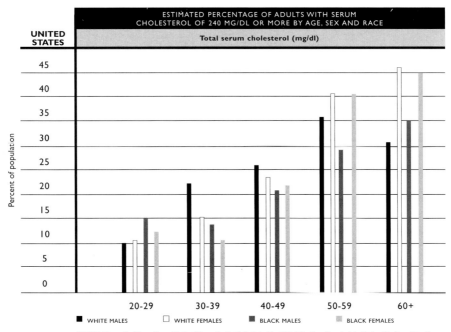

ESTIMATED PERCENTAGE OF ADULTS WITH SERUM CHOLESTEROL OF 240 MG/DL OR MORE BY AGE, SEX AND RACE		

UNITED STATES

Total serum cholesterol (mg/dl)

Percent of population

45
40
35
30
25
20
15
10
5
0

20-29   30-39   40-49   50-59   60+

■ WHITE MALES   □ WHITE FEMALES   ■ BLACK MALES   ▨ BLACK FEMALES

SOURCE: Centers for Disease Control/National Center for Health Statistics: Unpublished data from Phase I of the National Health and Nutrition Examination Survey III (Hanes III).

In order to reduce blood cholesterol, you should reduce the amount of dietary cholesterol consumed. Although the American Heart Association recommends a daily cholesterol intake of no more than 300 mg per day, the average American diet has been estimated to contain 500 – 1,000 mg per day.

Every 34 seconds an American dies
of cardiovascular disease.[31]

The reality is that the body does not need any extra cholesterol. So from a health standpoint, we are better off not consuming it at all. When we consume cholesterol, our cholesterol level goes up; when we cut back, the level drops. If we consume no cholesterol, little saturated fat, and exercise regularly, something wonderful happens: our cholesterol level drops significantly.

Meat, particularly organ meat (liver, kidney), and dairy products (milk, cream, cheese, butter, and ice cream) contain significant amounts of cholesterol. One cup of whole milk has 33 mg of cholesterol, while one egg yolk has 274 mg of cholesterol. The diet I am proposing is built around fruits, vegetables, grains, and legumes, none of which contain any cholesterol. Moreover, a number of plant foods, including almonds, cashews, whole grains, soybeans, corn, and some vegetable oils, contain important compounds called phytosterols and tocotrienols, which have been shown to prevent the absorption of cholesterol and thereby lower serum cholesterol levels.[32]

In addition to cholesterol, equal emphasis should be placed on dietary fat, particularly the saturated variety, the type that prevails in animal products. Research shows that eating less saturated fat may be the most important factor in reducing cholesterol levels and the risk of CHD. One reason is that saturated fat stimulates the production of cholesterol in the body. Conveniently though, in most cases, cholesterol and saturated fat come packaged together in the same foods. So, by eliminating animal products, you win both wars.

HYPERTENSION

An estimated 63 million Americans aged six and older have hypertension, more commonly known as high blood pressure.[33] Because there are no warning signs, unless we have our blood pressure checked periodically, it is unlikely we will be aware of it until it is critically high. In fact, about 35 percent of those who are hypertensive are unaware of the fact.[34] Hypertension is a risk factor for coronary heart disease, stroke, and heart attack. Research has also concluded that with every 10mm Hg increase in systolic blood pressure, there is a 9 percent increase in risk of impaired attention, concentration, memory, and judgment.[35]

Except in rare cases of adrenal gland or kidney disease, most cases of hypertension are called "essential," meaning they have no specific cause. However, we know of several factors that adversely affect blood pressure levels. They include a diet high in sodium, excessive alcohol consumption, smoking, and obesity.

Blood pressure is the measurement of force against the arterial walls during the contraction and resting phases of the heart. A blood pressure reading is given with two numbers, systolic and diastolic. The systolic represents the force during contraction and the diastolic represents the force between contractions, when the heart rests. A person is usually considered hypertensive if her blood pressure exceeds 140/90 mm of mercury (Hg).

One cause of hypertension is a high intake of dietary sodium. Animal-source foods such as milk, cheese, butter, beef jerky, hot dogs, and luncheon meats, as well as canned and frozen foods, contain enormous amounts of sodium. Table salt, composed of 60 percent chloride and 40 percent sodium, is another major source.

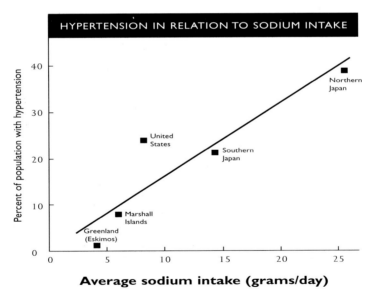

Average sodium intake (grams/day)

SOURCE: Brown, Judity E., *The Science of Human Nutrition*
(New York: HBJ, 1990): 362

Americans sprinkle an average of 2-3 teaspoons of salt on their food each day. Each teaspoon of table salt contains 2,000 mg of sodium.

Also, a diet high in fat and cholesterol will increase blood pressure in two additional ways. Such a diet increases the chance of atherosclerosis, the progressive accumulation of plaque narrowing the artery channel. Consequently, the flow of blood through the artery is met with greater resistance, and blood pressure rises. Dietary fat is also believed to influence blood pressure by causing the blood cells to clump together, thereby thickening the blood. A study that involved over 28,000 Seventh-Day Adventists found that high blood pressure was 75 percent more common among omnivores than vegetarians.

DIABETES

Current estimates are that diabetes affects the lives of about 20 million people in the United States, five million cases of which have not been diagnosed. This represents nearly a 50 percent increase in cases since 1983! About 300,000 people die annually from the disease and about 75 percent of these deaths are attributable to coronary heart disease that results from the condition. All told, the cost of medical treatment for the disease exceeds $18 billion.

There are two types of diabetes. Type I is known as insulin-dependent and Type II as non-insulin-dependent (sometimes referred to as adult-onset diabetes). The less common form, Type I (about 10 percent of all cases), usually occurs during youth, but may appear at any age when the pancreas becomes damaged and no longer produces the hormone insulin. Some pancreatic damage is believed to be due to a viral infection that damages the beta cells of the pancreas. Some individuals are genetically susceptible to the infection. Another theory (for which there is considerable evidence) considers the potential damage caused by the proteins in cow's milk. We will look more closely at this latter theory in Chapter Eleven.

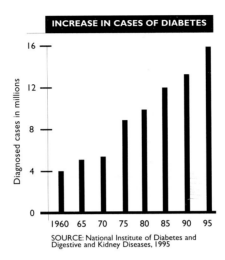

INCREASE IN CASES OF DIABETES

Diagnosed cases in millions

16
12
8
4
0

1960 65 70 75 80 85 90 95

SOURCE: National Institute of Diabetes and
Digestive and Kidney Diseases, 1995

Insulin is critical in the process of "fueling" the cells of the body. In order to function, the cells need a form of sugar that is derived from the foods we eat. Insulin is integral in presenting that sugar to the cells. When insulin is not present, the sugar remains circulating in the bloodstream. Without insulin, individuals have very little energy, and become ill easily. Other health problems associated with diabetes include elevated cholesterol levels, atherosclerosis, coronary heart disease, stroke, blindness, and capillary and nerve damage, severe cases of which require amputation of limbs.

To counter this problem, insulin-dependent diabetics require multiple, daily injections of insulin coupled with a restricted diet. Type I diabetes is a hereditary disease, and so diet does not play a role in its onset. Although diet may help control Type I diabetes, sadly, there is no cure.

Type II diabetes is far more common, accounting for about 90 percent of all cases. Here, insulin is present, but the body has difficulty in utilizing the hormone. In most Type II cases, injections are not necessary. It is believed that the cell receptors are desensitized to insulin and, as a result, insulin is improperly transported across cell membranes. In both cases, without treatment, glucose (blood sugar) that is not utilized builds up around the cells and stockpiles in the blood, raising blood glucose levels, and eventually overflowing into the urine.

Type II diabetes may ultimately be the result of obesity, excessive levels of body fat, and a sedentary lifestyle. In fact, over 80 percent of those with Type II diabetes are overweight, if not obese. Obesity, in turn, is most often the result of a diet of excessive fat intake and a sedentary lifestyle.

Like heart disease, Type II diabetes develops progressively over an extended period, usually without symptoms. Obesity, high body fat, and a sedentary lifestyle seem to decrease the number of effective insulin receptors. On the other hand, regular exercise, a low-fat, high-fiber diet, and weight loss tend to increase the number of cell insulin receptors. Therefore, Type II diabetes is preventable through proper nutrition, maintaining a healthy body weight, and regular exercise.

Diabetics will benefit greatly from the Revised American Diet because it is rich in complex carbohydrates and fiber, low in fat, and low in refined sugar.

Let's look more closely at these benefits.

1. By eating complex carbohydrates and other high-fiber foods, the assimilation of sugars into the bloodstream is more gradual than with refined foods. There is less of a chance of the sugar stockpiling in the blood when it is unable to cross the cellular membrane. There is also a reduction in the level of insulin needed to balance blood sugar levels.

2. By consuming foods low in fat, insulin function improves significantly because fat interferes with the function of insulin, specifically its ability to bind with the hungry cells and deliver their needed sugar.

3. By eliminating cholesterol from their diet, diabetics' risk of developing atherosclerosis is reduced significantly.

4. By bringing about effective and lasting weight loss, the Revised American Diet will be both preventive as well as corrective. Since being overweight is a risk factor

for diabetes, by not becoming overweight, one will reduce the chance of developing adult-onset diabetes. Those who already have diabetes find such a diet actually reduces their symptoms, and, in some cases, may even eliminate the disease.

OBESITY

It is a sad fact that America leads the world in obesity. Individuals are considered obese when they are 30 percent over the "desirable" weight for their age, sex, and height. This condition has reached epidemic proportions in the United States. Current estimates from the National Health and Nutrition Examination Survey indicate that currently 47 million American adults are obese, and that by the end of 1996, 34 percent of the United States population will be obese. The hazards of obesity are numerous, and include: excessive strain on the lower back, hips and legs; crowding of internal organs (of particular concern are the lungs, which cannot fully expand, resulting in shallow breathing); increased resistance to insulin, thereby increasing the chance of developing Type II diabetes; increased risk of developing hypertension, heart disease, heart attack, and stroke; and the development of various types of cancers. While obesity has not been a primary risk factor in breast cancer, an important study in the medical journal *Cancer* demonstrates that "body fat distribution significantly increases the risk for breast cancer, and affects the prognosis after the diagnosis of breast cancer." Specifically, the study finds that women who carry fat primarily in their upper bodies (android obesity), as opposed to their lower bodies (gynoid obesity), are at heightened risk. The study also showed that those women who reduced their body weight by approximately 12 pounds effectively reduced their risk by 45 percent. There is also evidence that obesity increases risk of uterine cancer in premenopausal women.

Most recently, researchers at Boston University School of Public Health have concluded that obese women are more likely to give birth to babies with anencephaly and spina bifida.

The primary causes of obesity are excessive dietary fat consumption and lack of exercise.

OSTEOPOROSIS

Osteoporosis is a disease that results in an increasing narrowing and frailty of the bones, ultimately resulting in fractures. It is a significant problem for Americans, particularly women. Each year, approximately 1.5 million osteoporosis-related bone fractures are reported, about 500,000 of which occur in postmenopausal women. While osteoporosis has traditionally been associated with inadequate calcium intake, substantial evidence implicates as strong causes excessive protein and phosphorus consumption, caffeine consumption, smoking, and sedentary living. In the second part of this book, we will see how weight-bearing exercises decrease the risk of this disease. Now let's look at the role diet plays in its onset.

Scientific studies document that an excessively high-protein diet (particularly animal protein) leads to a negative calcium balance, and, in turn, serious risk for osteoporosis.[36] Yet Americans keep hearing the same message, "Drink your milk, eat your yogurt, enjoy more cheese." Beyond this, the business of selling calcium supplement tablets is booming. In 1995, over $200 million worth were consumed by Americans who hoped to prevent a calcium deficiency.

The truth is, it is important to look at how much calcium one retains, rather than what one consumes. When we compare worldwide rates of osteoporosis, we see that the disease is relatively rare in places where protein is consumed in moderate amounts. Conversely, countries with the highest rates of osteoporosis (Norway, Sweden, and Denmark) also have the highest intakes of animal proteins. Why is this? High levels of protein result in more acidic blood. In an effort to buffer this acid and achieve a more appropriate blood balance, the body utilizes calcium, eventually drawing on the calcium stored in the bones, a process known as "calcium leaching."

In one study, individuals consuming excess protein were found to have a negative calcium balance of 137 mg per day. Estimates were that, at this rate, the annual rate of loss could reach 50 grams of calcium with the potential for a skeletal mass loss of 4 percent a year. Another important finding in this study was the fact that, regardless of how much dietary calcium was increased (through calcium-rich foods or supplements), it could not compensate for the calcium losses as long as subjects remained on an excessively high-protein diet. In other words, as long as one's protein intake remains excessively high, one can swallow all the calcium supplement tablets one wishes and still suffer a calcium deficiency.[37]

To illustrate this further, consider the native Inuits. Their diet, composed primarily of fish, walrus, and whale, provides them with enormous amounts of calcium (upwards of 2,000 mg a day) because of the bones contained in the fish meat they eat. Such a calcium intake is over twice the United States RDA. Therefore, if more calcium is better, we should expect osteoporosis to be unheard of among the Inuits. Unfortunately, the truth is just the opposite. The Inuits have one of the highest rates of osteoporosis in the world; correspondingly, they also have one of the highest intakes of protein in the world (300-400 grams a day). Obviously, more calcium in one's diet is not necessarily better.

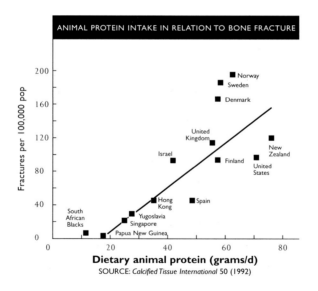

SOURCE: *Calcified Tissue International* 50 (1992)

ANIMAL PROTEIN AND OSTEOPOROSIS

Two factors make animal protein more calcium-costly than plant protein. As mentioned, excessive protein intake leads to greater urinary calcium losses. With excess protein the blood becomes more acidic. To buffer this acid rise the body relies on calcium, which it may leach from the bones. Compounding the problem is the fact that animal protein has more sulfur-containing amino acids which tend to increase calcium losses. Further, animal foods contain higher levels of phosphorus that may interfere with calcium absorption. Phosphorus is an important component to health, but in levels disproportionate to calcium (such as in cow's milk), it may bind with calcium in the digestive tract and sharply reduce its absorption. Numerous studies confirm that this process of "calcium leaching" is more likely to occur with the consumption of animal protein than with vegetable protein.[38] One such study was conducted at the University of Texas Southwestern Medical Center. In this study, human subjects were given equal amounts of protein, first from animal foods, then from a strict vegan diet. Calcium losses were measurably higher during the animal-diet phase of the study.

Plant-based foods have more moderate levels of protein, less sulfur-containing amino acids, and a better calcium to phosphorus ratio, making their calcium easier to absorb and their protein less of a threat to the body's calcium stores (bones).

Many people fear that if they don't drink milk and consume milk products, they will not be getting enough calcium, protein, or vitamin D, their bones will disintegrate, and their teeth will fall out. It's no accident that this fear exists. A great deal of advertising on the part of milk producers, as well as advice from misguided healthcare professionals, has played a big role in reinforcing this fear. After all these years of being told that we must drink the milk of another species to maintain strong bones, the reality is that no legitimate research supports this myth. On the contrary, volumes of research have continued to demonstrate that those who ingest large amounts of milk are at higher risk of osteoporosis, obesity, elevated cholesterol, heart disease, and kidney stones.

mg per 1 cup	CALCIUM CONTENT OF VARIOUS FOODS
	VEGETABLES
245 mg	SPINACH
197 mg	TURNIP GREENS
177 mg	BROCCOLI
148 mg	COLLARD GREENS
147 mg	DANDELION GREENS
115 mg	RHUBARB
104 mg	MUSTARD GREENS
102 mg	SWISS CHARD
94 mg	KALE
57 mg	ONION
	LEGUMES
175 mg	SOYBEANS
128 mg	NAVY BEANS
95 mg	PEAS
90 mg	GREAT NORTHERN BEANS
86 mg	PINTO BEANS
55 mg	LIMA BEANS
47 mg	BLACK BEANS
37 mg	LENTILS
	ANIMAL FOODS
115 mg	MILK
16 mg	BEEF STEAK
14 mg	EGG
14 mg	CHICKEN
11 mg	PORK
10 mg	TUNA
	NUTS AND SEEDS
245 mg	ALMONDS
209 mg	HAZELNUTS
131 mg	PISTACHIOS
126 mg	SUNFLOWER SEEDS
110 mg	SESAME SEEDS

Several studies have been conducted on societies that do not consume any dairy products to see if their members are at any greater risk for a calcium deficiency and subsequent weak bones and teeth. In one such study, elderly African women who consumed no milk or dairy products were examined. While conventional wisdom would predict that these women would be frail and at heightened risk for bone fracture, the reality was very different. All of them had strong bones and teeth and not one showed a calcium deficiency. While the average American consumes in excess of 1,000 mg of calcium a day, the African women consumed approximately 500 mg daily and only from vegetable, grain, and legume sources.[39] These women have a positive calcium balance because they retain the calcium they consume. Contrary to what one might have heard, leafy greens, vegetables, legumes, raw nuts, and seeds contain plenty of calcium.

Although the current recommended daily intake for calcium is actually 800-1,200 mg, it is based upon a diet that is excessive in protein. When protein intake is reduced to modest levels, and protein is derived from vegetables, legumes, and grains, an intake closer to 500 mg of calcium becomes adequate.

As you can see, there is a potent relationship between the foods we eat and our level of health. So why are so few of us familiar with the risks outlined above? One reason is that those who are most likely to influence our health – physicians and other healthcare providers – are themselves mostly uninformed about nutrition. Like the patients they treat, most medical doctors have adopted the common food myths and prescribe eating habits that will likely ensure that their patients continue to return. Yet medical doctors cannot be blamed entirely for their ignorance. It has been found that of the 125 medical schools in this country, only 30 require anything more than three hours in basic nutrition for their graduates. Unfortunately, the emphasis in medical school is placed on treating illnesses once they have developed rather than on preventing them from occurring. This is unfair to both doctors and patients. In addition, physicians are the target of a pharmaceutical industry that spends some $5 billion annually promoting products that are designed for treatment rather than prevention of illness.

By altering our currently unhealthy diets, each of us can do much to prevent numerous degenerative illnesses before they ever begin to ravage our bodies. With the assistance of such organizations as the Physicians Committee for Responsible Medicine, this truth is beginning to reach both healthcare providers and the general public.

THE MACRONUTRIENTS

When Health is absent, Wisdom cannot reveal itself, Art cannot become manifest,
Strength cannot be exerted, Wealth is useless and Reason is powerless.
– Herophiles

While people are now more familiar with the various nutrients than ever, there is still a great deal of confusion about the role each of these nutrients plays in our diet. This confusion has contributed to the poor dietary choices made by the general public. Before we look at the Revised American Diet, we need to examine the following nutrients: proteins, carbohydrates, fats, and water. Following is an overview of these nutrients that will demystify their particular dietary roles and help to dispel the many myths that have evolved around their necessity in the diet.

PROTEIN

Dietary protein is chiefly responsible for building, maintaining, and repairing the muscles (the proteins actin and myosin) and connective tissues (the proteins collagen, elastin, and keratin) of the body. We are made of protein; our muscles, organs, and even our hair has been constructed from protein. Proteins are also the foundation for the synthesis of hormones, enzymes, and antibodies.

The "building blocks" of protein are the amino acids. They are divided into two groups. The first group consists of the non-essential amino acids, which the body is capable of manufacturing by itself. The second group consists of the essential amino acids, those that the body cannot synthesize and, therefore, must derive from food sources.

Unfortunately, Americans seem to be preoccupied with their consumption of protein. The protein intake in the American diet is quite adequate, and sometimes superfluous. In fact, studies have shown that in most cases the amount of protein consumed greatly exceeds the level necessary to support muscle development. The latest U. S. Department of Agriculture survey reveals that the recommended allowance for protein is exceeded in all age categories. In their quest for more protein, most people rely primarily on foods of animal origin – foods that naturally contain large amounts of fat and cholesterol, and that are strongly associated with disease. Three popular myths associated with protein play a key role in its overconsumption.

ESSENTIAL AND NON-ESSENTIAL AMINO ACIDS

ESSENTIAL	NON-ESSENTIAL
Histidine	Asparagine
Isoleucine	Alanine
Leucine	Aspartic acid
Lysine	Arginine
Methionine	Cysteine
Phenylalanine	Cystine
Threonine	Glutamine
Tryptophan	Glutamic acid
Valine	Glycine
	Hydroxylysine
	Hydroxyproline
	Tyrosine
	Proline
	Serine

MYTH #1

The first myth is that protein provides the body with energy. *"The more protein I eat, the more energy I'll have."* I have often overheard people say things like, "I'm exhausted, I really need some protein," or "I have to have a protein shake before I exercise today." Somehow, somebody got the idea that protein "energizes" the body.

As previously mentioned, out of the three primary nutrients (fat, carbohydrates, and protein) protein is the last and least-efficient source from which muscular energy is generated. Carbohydrates are the chief form of muscle fuel, followed by fat, and finally, if necessary, protein. The body spares protein so that it can be utilized foremost in the construction and maintenance of body tissues.

MYTH #2

Another myth surrounding protein is that when it comes to muscle growth and athletic performance, more is better. Protein "bombardment" is popular among athletes because it has been suggested that athletes and those who exercise with greater intensity (particularly those who are attempting to build larger muscles) have an increased protein requirement. For this reason many athletes will increase protein intake by two times or more the recommended daily intake, either through large amounts of protein-rich food (e.g., protein shakes), or through supplemental amino acids. In my experience working with athletes, it is not uncommon to hear of a diet consisting of 125-200 grams of protein a day or more. Of course this far exceeds the suggested daily protein intake of approximately 60 grams. The truth is that the body does not utilize this excess protein. In other words, just because a person consumes more protein doesn't mean the body is going to manufacture more muscle. Instead, the body, specifically the kidneys and liver, must work overtime to get rid of the excess protein load, and, as a consequence, the kidneys and liver may become enlarged and prematurely age.

I once read an article in a popular fitness magazine in which a television star and athlete was interviewed about his diet. This individual extolled the virtues of a "mega-high-protein" diet, and explained how a regular breakfast for him consisted of approximately 13 egg whites. While this man is intelligent enough to remove the yolks from this enormous quantity of eggs and thus spare himself nearly 3,000 mg of cholesterol and 78 grams of fat, he clearly remains a victim of what I call the "great protein myth." Also, in an encyclopedic fitness book, the author advised readers to have many small meals a day in an effort to consume as much protein as possible. By his prescription, each meal should contain 40-50 grams of protein, thereby providing a highly excessive 250 grams of protein daily, equal to over 400 percent of the RDA for protein. Contrary to what most athletes and many of their coaches have been led to believe, and what many food supplement products suggest to the consumer, there is not a speck of research to support the theory that larger quantities of protein create larger and stronger muscles!

MYTH #3

The third myth is that protein is only available from animal-source foods. This simply is not so. These myths have played a big part in the overconsumption of protein, particularly animal proteins. Several diseases and conditions are strongly linked to this overconsumption, including osteoporosis, kidney disease, and obesity.

ANIMAL PROTEIN AND OSTEOPOROSIS

In Chapter Five, Diseases and Diet, we looked closely at the relationship between excessive protein and the increase in risk of osteoporosis. It was shown that animal protein in particular accelerates calcium losses, resulting in frail bones and increased risk of bone fracture. If you are not reading these chapters sequentially, you may wish to refer back to that section now.

ANIMAL PROTEIN AND KIDNEY DISEASE

The excessive protein intake from a diet based upon animal products places tremendous strain on the kidneys, and can, in the long run, contribute to permanent kidney damage. Today nearly 20 million Americans suffer from kidney damage and some 200,000 live with the assistance of an artificial kidney machine. When patients cut back on their protein consumption, they not only slow the progression of their disease, but they may avoid dialysis altogether.

ANIMAL PROTEIN AND EXCESSIVE WEIGHT

Excessive protein in the diet, particularly animal protein, may also be a key factor in the number of overweight people in America. The reason for this is that the protein foods most commonly included in the diet — derived from animal sources (meat, cheese, and milk, for example) — also happen to be very high in saturated fat. I don't believe that most people set out to consume a high-fat diet. Most people erroneously believe that they can only satisfy their body's protein needs by getting their protein from these conventional sources, which happen to contain a great deal of fat. But our protein needs are not nearly as great as we have been led to believe, and we have many foods that can satisfy our protein requirement. In fact, about two-thirds of the world's population survive quite well and meet their protein requirement while consuming little, if any, animal foods. Consequently, they are relatively free of heart disease and other effects of a diet rich in animal products.

AREN'T PLANT FOODS INFERIOR?

Plant-source proteins are sometimes called "incomplete," which only means they are lacking or low in one or more amino acids and, therefore, ideally should be combined with other complementary protein sources to form a complete protein. As an example, rice, a highly nutritious food, happens to be high in the amino acid methionine, yet low in the amino acid lysine. Beans, however, are high in lysine and low in methionine. Therefore, these two foods complement each other. Another complementation is peanuts and bread. When combined in a peanut butter sandwich, they form a complete protein, as much as found in a piece of meat or fish. The reality is that complementary proteins have been a mainstay of numerous traditional diets around the world, but not because people were necessarily concerned about "complete proteins."

Below is a list of complementary proteins eaten in various regions of the world:

LATIN AMERICA

Rice and beans

Corn tortilla and beans

MIDDLE EAST

Bulgur wheat and chickpeas

Pita bread and hummus

INDIA

Lentils and rice

ASIA

Soy foods and rice

Recent research has confirmed that because the body has its own pool of amino acids to draw upon, precision and timing in the consumption of complementary proteins are unnecessary.[40] In other words, if one had a deficient diet during a particular period, the body could draw upon its protein pool to compensate. While there are numerous vegetable-source proteins that complement each other, one does not have to eat two complementary proteins simultaneously. They can be eaten at the same meal, at another meal that day, or even the next day.

GETTING ENOUGH PROTEIN: IT'S EASIER THAN YOU MIGHT THINK

In reality, as long as one eats a wide variety of foods and takes in a sufficient number of calories, one is bound to obtain all of the essential amino acids, because nearly all foods contain some protein. Results of the Health and Nutrition Examination Survey (HANES) indicate that a protein deficiency is in fact relatively rare, and is more often than not the result of a total calorie deficiency rather than a failure to eat enough proteins. Further, a U.S. Department of Agriculture study reveals that even on a strict vegetarian diet, Americans consumed 150 percent of their protein needs! The following list shows the percentage of calories as protein in various plant-source foods.

percent	PERCENT OF PROTEIN IN PLANT FOODS
	VEGETABLES
49%	SPINACH
47%	BROCCOLI
40%	CAULIFLOWER
38%	MUSHROOMS
34%	PARSLEY
34%	LETTUCE
28%	ZUCCHINI
26%	GREEN BEANS
24%	CUCUMBER
21%	CELERY
18%	TOMATOES
16%	ONIONS
11%	POTATOES
	LEGUMES
43%	TOFU
30%	GREEN PEAS
29%	LENTILS
26%	KIDNEY BEANS
26%	NAVY BEANS
23%	CHICK PEAS
	GRAINS
20%	RYE
17%	WHEAT
16%	OATMEAL
15%	BUCKWHEAT
11%	BARLEY
8%	BROWN RICE

FATS

With all of the negative press regarding dietary fat, some people seem determined to eliminate every trace of fat from their diet. I have had people tell me, "Oh, I don't eat any fat at all." The reality is that a "zero-fat diet" is next to impossible. One reason is that at least some fat exists in a wide variety of foods. Furthermore, contrary to what some people might believe, such a diet is undesirable. Humans simply can't survive without dietary fat.

In our determination to rid our diets of excess fats, some of us may have forgotten the important role fat plays in human health. For example, fats provide storage for and transport the fat-soluble vitamins. They are essential to proper growth and development. Body fat (adipose tissue) acts as an insulator to help reduce heat loss in colder temperatures and provides protection from injury by cushioning vital organs.

Like the essential amino acids, certain fats cannot be manufactured by the body and therefore must be derived from the foods we eat. These include the Omega-3 and Omega-6 essential fatty acids (EFAs). Among their many contributions, the EFAs are important to the maintenance of hair, skin, blood vessels, nerves, and cellular integrity. Omega-3s also assist in immunity to illness. They do this by stimulating the production of prostaglandins, hormone-like substances that not only regulate immune function, but dilate blood vessels and prevent blood platelet stickiness.[41] There is also evidence that the Omega-3s help control triglyceride and cholesterol levels.[42]

While most of us get plenty of Omega-6s in our diet, those who follow the Standard American Diet risk developing an Omega-3 deficiency. This is because the SAD is often lacking in Omega-3 sources such as broccoli, spinach, soy, and legumes.

So, the question is not whether we should ingest dietary fat, but instead, what variety of fat, and in what quantities, will best promote health? While we will look at the variety of fats in detail to better understand how they act in the body and what effects they may have on our health, I want to assure you that the Revised American Diet proposed in this book will not require you to calculate fat grams and percentages. The beauty of the Revised American Diet is that it eliminates the need for this tedious preoccupation. The Revised American Diet makes it possible for you to obtain all of the necessary fats that your body needs, including the essential fatty acids, while helping you avoid those fats that compromise your health. Let's look more closely.

Fats are composed of carbon, hydrogen, and oxygen. A concentrated source of energy, a gram of fat yields more than twice the number of calories (nine) as either a gram of protein or carbohydrate (four). This characteristic increases the likelihood of an excessive caloric intake when fats make up a large part of the diet.

There are three primary types of naturally occurring fat: saturated, mono-unsaturated, and polyunsaturated. We will also look at two additional fats, the trans-fats, which are created through a process called hydrogenation, and a synthetic fat called Olestra.

SATURATED FATS

Saturated fats tend to be solid at room temperature. If you were to examine a saturated fat molecule, you would find that it contains the maximum amount of hydrogen atoms it can hold, hence it is "saturated" with hydrogen. Saturated fats are concentrated in foods of animal origin such as beef, pork, chicken, fish, cheese, milk, and butter. They are also highly concentrated in a few vegetable oils, including coconut oil, palm oil, and palm kernel oil.

MONOUNSATURATED FATS

Monounsaturated fats are liquid at room temperature. If you were to compare a monounsaturated fat molecule with the polyunsaturated variety, you would find that it is missing a hydrogen atom from both adjoining carbon atoms. This necessitates a double bond between carbon atoms.

they eat. Yet, even when animal products are eliminated entirely from the diet, some people will rely quite heavily on the use of vegetable oils. Furthermore, they may rely on oils that have been highly processed and mishandled. While there are some vegetable oils that are more healthful than others, and even a few that are used therapeutically because of their rich EFA content, I recommend that any vegetable oil be used sparingly. If used, vegetable oils should be fresh, preferably organic, and properly cared for. Following is a list of the oils that I believe are most healthful, as well as guidelines for properly caring for vegetable oils.

Borage, Black Currant, and Evening Primrose oils

Borage, black current, and evening primrose oils not only are rich in EFAs, but also contain gamma-linoleic acid (GLA), about 24 percent, 18 percent, and 9 percent respectively. Normally, the body synthesizes GLA from linoleic acid (Omega-6), but viral infections and other diseases, and a high intake of processed fats (especially TFAs), cholesterol, and sugar, as well as diabetes, can impair this conversion. Borage, black currant and evening primrose oils have been used therapeutically to treat premenstrual symptoms, arthritis, inflammation, and immune disorders. All three of these oils are available in capsule form.

Flaxseed Oil

While flaxseed oil contains about 20 percent Omega-6 EFAs, it is one of the richest sources of the Omega-3s (57 percent). For this reason it is sometimes used as a supplemental oil. The consumption of both flaxseeds and their oil has been associated with a reduction in LDL (bad) cholesterol,[48] improved immune function,[49] and reduced risk of blood platelet aggregation.[50] Treatment for long-term amenorrhea (cessation of the menstrual cycle) sometimes includes supplementation with one to two tablespoons of fresh flaxseed oil taken daily in conjunction with 400 units of vitamin E to protect against oxidation. Two Scottish researchers, Peter O. Behan and Wilhelmina M.H. Behan, of Glasgow University, have used Omega-3 supplementation to treat depression and lack of concentration. Other physicians have successfully used Omega-3 supplementation to treat yeast conditions, muscular fatigue, and inflammation.

Flaxseed oil has a pleasant nutty taste that most people enjoy. However, some people prefer to buy flaxseed oil that has been encapsulated. Another option is to buy whole flaxseeds and grind them in a coffee grinder when you wish to use them. In this ground form they can be added to salads and vegetable dishes, and their EFA content will be well absorbed.

Flaxseed oil is found refrigerated at natural foods markets (both bottled and in capsule form). In capsule form, flaxseed oil is packaged together with vitamin E and beta carotene to protect it from oxidation. If bottled, purchase it only in small amounts so that it will be used before it can turn rancid. Flaxseed oil should always be kept tightly sealed and refrigerated, and should never be heated.

Hempseed Oil

Contrary to what one might expect, this oil is legal. Derived from the seeds of the marijuana plant, hempseed oil contains a fair amount of Omega-3 EFAs (about 20 percent) and is particularly rich in Omega-6 EFAs (about 60 percent). It has a wonderful peanut-like flavor. Currently, hempseed oil can be difficult to find. However, soon it should be available in better natural foods markets. Like flaxseed oil, the nutritional quality of this oil is highly vulnerable to heat and light. Therefore it is found refrigerated in dark plastic containers and should never be heated. In the Appendix you will find information for special ordering this oil.

Olive Oil

While olive oil is low in EFAs, it has a very favorable fat profile, as monounsaturates account for about 75 percent of its fat content. Besides its wonderful taste, virgin olive oil is the only mass-marketed oil that has not been refined or heated to temperatures above 150 degrees (302°F), and therefore, it retains most of its nutrient value. When shopping for olive oil be sure that the label says "virgin."

Unfortunately, most of the oils available to consumers have not been well cared for prior to reaching market. Usually they are highly refined and subjected to many processes that compromise their nutritional value. Oils in general are extremely vulnerable to light, oxygen, and heat, and the more they are exposed to these elements, the more they degenerate into unhealthy products.

When we examine the oils we bring home from the market, they seem clear and pure. However, the handling of oils, from the extraction of the oil from the seed to the packaging and storage of oils in our homes, can have serious consequences, and may well accelerate the development of nutrient-deficient and rancid oil.

Some oils have been extracted with the use of toxic solvents such as hexane, the residues of which stay with the oil. This is why oils that have been "expeller-pressed" are preferable. Most all mass-marketed oils have been subjected to processes of defoaming, degumming, and deodorizing, as well as heated to excessively high temperatures. These processes and others not only accelerate the degeneration of oils, they also remove many of the healthful components of the oil such as phytosterols, chlorophyll, beta carotene, and vitamin E. Once the oils are brought home from the market they are subjected to further mishandling. For instance, excess light can produce free radicals, ketones, and other toxic components. Light also makes oil more vulnerable to oxygen, which ages oil quickly and deteriorates the vital essential fatty acids. Heat is the most detrimental element to which oils are exposed because it changes the molecular structure of the fat.

The best oils (the most biologically active) are those that are unrefined and that have been derived from organically grown crops. Non-organic oils are likely to contain dangerous pesticide residues. All oil should be purchased in green or brown glass bottles, or, in the case of flaxseed and hempseed oils, black plastic bottles. They should be sealed tightly after use and stored in the refrigerator.

Again, research continues to confirm that the best sources of fat are vegetables and grains, and, in limited amounts, raw nuts and seeds. The guidelines for the Revised American Diet suggest avoiding animal products entirely. By doing so, you will be eliminating from your diet not only the primary source of unwanted saturated fats, but also all dietary cholesterol.

Additionally, you should exclude foods that contain the highly saturated coconut, palm, and palm kernel oils (found in many baked goods and most movie theater popcorn). Be sure to avoid foods that contain hydrogenated or partially hydrogenated oil, which are sources of TFAs. While you should always check the ingredient label to be sure, the most likely culprits are commercial sandwich breads, tortillas, cookies, crackers, microwave popcorn, margarine, and solid vegetable shortening.

CARBOHYDRATES

The chief function of carbohydrates is to provide the body with fuel. Carbohydrates provide energy, not only for muscles but for the vital functions of the brain and nervous system. The cells of the nervous system are dependent on a regular supply of carbohydrates. The brain utilizes nearly 500 calories from carbohydrates every day! This is why it always amazes me when I hear of people on very low or no-carbohydrate fad diets. What they are doing is depriving the brain, as well as the rest of the body, of its chief source of energy, and the inevitable result is an individual "on edge." These people become nervous, forgetful, irritable, and sluggish. Yet one doesn't need to follow a fad diet to avoid carbohydrates. The Standard American Diet itself is significantly deficient in this nutrient because beef, pork, chicken, and fish have almost no carbohydrates. When people make the transition to the Revised American Diet (RAD), one of the first things they notice is the incredible abundance of energy they enjoy because they are discarding a carbohydrate-deficient diet in favor of one that is centered upon complex carbohydrates.

When the body ingests carbohydrates, it first converts a portion into glucose (blood sugar), which the liver will be responsible for releasing into the bloodstream for fuel. The remaining portion is converted into glycogen and stored in the muscles and liver. Fat and protein can be used for energy if necessary, but both must first be converted in a process that requires energy, taxes the liver and kidneys, and creates excessive metabolic waste. Carbohydrates are our most efficient source of accessible energy, and our bodies naturally crave them!

Carbohydrates, also known as sugars, are formed of carbon, oxygen, and hydrogen. They are classified by the number of carbon atoms they contain and by how simple forms are combined into more complex forms. For instance, a carbohydrate designated "simple" is a monosaccharide (mono meaning "single" and saccharide meaning "sugar"). If two monosaccharides are combined they form a disaccharide. Several monosaccharides or disaccharides linked together form what are called polysaccharides (poly meaning "many"). Polysaccharides are commonly referred to as complex carbohydrates.

Examples of simple carbohydrates are white sugar or white flour. Examples of complex carbohydrates are whole grains, vegetables, and legumes.

Because simple carbohydrates tend to be void of important vitamins, minerals, and fiber, they are often said to offer "empty calories." Complex carbohydrates, on the other hand, tend to be high in vitamins, minerals, and fiber. The majority of your carbohydrate calories should come from the complex variety.

One problem with simple carbohydrates such as table sugar and corn syrup is that they are absorbed rapidly by the body and quickly raise the blood sugar level. Complex carbohydrates are absorbed much more slowly (usually over a period of several hours) and affect the blood sugar level at a more gradual rate. Lower-quality carbohydrates are found in foods that often are tempting, but hold little nutritional value, such as chocolate, cookies, and candy. When the body ingests these refined carbohydrates, higher than normal levels of insulin are released by the pancreas in order to contend with the rapidly elevated blood sugar level. Often, the quick release of insulin will quickly remove too much blood sugar, resulting in a significant drop in energy. This is a familiar experience to almost everyone. You've hit rock bottom. You have no energy. So you reach for a candy bar and devour it. Your energy level skyrockets. You feel as though you could lift a car! Then, usually within seven to ten minutes, you are worse off than before, your energy severely depressed; you have "come down." You probably feel like eating sweets again to get the "high," so you might reach for another dose of quick energy. It's a vicious cycle. You can avoid this seesaw experience simply by eating more fresh vegetables, whole grains, legumes, and fruits. These foods provide you with a balanced source of energy, and you won't find yourself continually feeling "low."

AREN'T CARBOHYDRATES FATTENING?

Many people are under the erroneous assumption that carbohydrates are a high-fat food source. On the contrary, carbohydrates are typically very low in fat. What can make carbohydrates fattening, however, are the sauces and toppings that often accompany them. For example, a six-ounce portion of linguine is a wonderful source of low-fat complex carbohydrates (if the pasta is made with no egg). However, one might decide to cover that pasta with an Alfredo cream sauce.

Baked potatoes, another wonderfully low-fat source of complex carbohydrates, can be seriously fattened up with the addition of a few tablespoons of sour cream, a little butter, and some bacon bits. So remember, it's not carbohydrates that are fattening, it's what we commonly put on top of them.

An added benefit of a diet rich in carbohydrates is a greater sense of well-being. Research conducted at the Massachusetts Institute of Technology has revealed that as carbohydrate intake is increased, so is the level of the neurotransmitter called serotonin. Serotonin has been found to promote a relaxed state, enhance the quality of sleep, and may improve concentration.

FIBER

Although fiber is classified as a form of carbohydrate, unlike other carbohydrates it is not absorbed through the intestinal wall and, therefore, is non-caloric. Fiber has been found to be helpful in the prevention of vascular disease and colon cancer and plays an important role in weight control. Moreover, those whose diets are high in fiber have a significantly lower incidence of gastrointestinal disorders such as diverticulitis, irritable colon, hemorrhoids, gallstones, and constipation.

Constipation is a major problem in the United States. Spend a couple of hours in front of the television and you'll be amazed by the number of products being touted as the cure for irregularity. Here is yet another example of how we typically address the symptoms rather than the cause.

Like most of the conditions mentioned thus far, constipation is largely the result of a diet centered on animal products. If you listen carefully to the advertisers of constipation cures, you'll hear them say that their products increase fiber intake. On a vegetarian diet you will take in an abundance of naturally occurring fiber and have no need for such products.

Fiber increases bowel motility, which in turn reduces transit time in the intestine. Reduced transit time means you will not only feel good, but also, there is a reduction in the chances for bacteria and other toxins to be retained in the intestines, where they might cause digestive problems and possible breakdown of the walls of the intestines, rendering the entire area more susceptible to cancer.

Because fiber is bound to digestible carbohydrates, the absorption of glucose is slowed down, reducing the need for secretions of insulin and allowing for a more balanced blood sugar level. It's also been found that water-soluble fibers chelate, or combine with, bile acids in the presence of cholesterol. As the supply of bile acids is reduced, the gallbladder synthesizes more, and in doing so removes more cholesterol from the bloodstream. This helps to reduce serum cholesterol levels.

Finally, because high-fiber foods are characteristically low in fat and provide bulk and therefore greater satiety, weight control is made easier with a fiber-rich diet.

In his excellent book *Immune Power*, Jon D. Kaiser, M.D., explains that fiber has the effect of "stimulating immune-enhancing cells called Peyer's patches found in the lining of the intestines. When stimulated, these cells help activate and strengthen the immune system by producing antibodies, which are the body's first line of defense against disease in the intestinal tract."[51]

While the National Cancer Institute recommends a daily fiber intake of 25-35 grams per day, studies continue to confirm the more fiber the better. Since the average American diet is estimated to contain only 11 grams a day, an increase to 30, of course, is a significant improvement. What we see, however, is that in those countries where diet-related diseases are lowest, fiber intake ranges from at least 33 grams to as high as 70 grams a day.

Although fiber itself does not provide the body with any energy, the foods it's contained within are usually abundant in complex carbohydrates, vitamins, and minerals! It really is no wonder that the SAD diet lacks fiber to such a degree: about two-thirds of its calories come from animal products, all of which offer little or no fiber.

	EXAMPLES OF FIBER-RICH FOODS
FRUITS	Apples, bananas, berries, cantaloupe, grapefruit, guava, mangoes, oranges, pineapple, papaya, pears.
VEGETABLES	Artichokes, broccoli, Brussel sprouts, carrots, corn, cauliflower, kale, potatoes, spinach, squash.
WHOLE GRAINS	Whole-wheat bread, muffins, bagels, and tortillas. Bran, bran-muffins, oatmeal, shredded wheat cereal, whole grain pasta, bulgar wheat, buckwheat, barley, quinoa, amaranth, millet, triticale, popcorn, rice cakes.
LEGUMES	Black beans, lima beans, kidney beans, navy beans, yellow, red, and green lentils, pinto beans, split peas, black-eyed peas, fava beans.

WATER

Water is indisputably the most important and predominant nutrient in your body. While you could survive for up to a month without food, you would perish in only days without water. Three-quarters of the human body weight is made up of water, so it is no wonder that we must constantly replenish our water supply in order to keep the body functioning properly. Water assists in many vital functions. It helps in the assimilation of foods and vitamins, carries nutrients and oxygen to the cells, and acts as a vehicle for the removal of bodily wastes. Therefore, water is a purifier. Probably the most important job water has in the body is regulating body temperature.

While it is recommended that the average person consume between eight and ten glasses of water each day, depending on diet and daily activities, regular exercise increases one's water needs because of the amount of water lost through perspiration. An individual can perspire as much as a quart of water per hour while training on a hot day. During exercise, our muscles generate heat, causing the body temperature to rise. In a very efficient process, heat from the muscles is removed by water present in the bloodstream and brought to the skin surface, where it is released by way of perspiration. As this process continues, the body eventually becomes dehydrated and is no longer able to effectively cool itself. In a state of dehydration, the amount of water normally contained in the blood drops low enough to create a drop in blood volume. In response to this drop, the body automatically constricts the blood vessels leading to the skin, serving to prevent a drop in blood pressure. You probably guessed the next phase. That's right. With a reduction of blood reaching the skin comes a reduction of heat being dissipated through the skin. The result? You overheat! And contrary to what we assume, thirst is not an accurate indicator of our water needs. You can avoid this risk simply by keeping your body well hydrated as you exercise.

By no means should you try to consume a large quantity of water all at once. It's not only difficult, but for some, it's sickening. The best method is to consume six to eight glasses of water a day even if you are not exercising. Prepare a large pitcher of water with a little fresh lemon squeezed into it, and over the course of a day, try to drink a glass or two every couple of hours. At work, simply keep bottled water close at hand. Before a workout, it's a good idea to drink about one cup of water. Then, every 10-15 minutes (depending on how vigorously you are exercising) consume another three to four ounces. Remember, you needn't be hot to lose water. The body loses water through the vapor of breath. In cold weather, the kidneys increase urine production, which also contributes to dehydration.

WHAT'S IN THE WATER YOU DRINK?

We have established the great need our bodies have for water, yet where we get that water from is another concern. No longer can we turn on the kitchen faucet and assume we are getting safely treated water. The average municipal water source is loaded with toxic contaminants including asbestos, lead, cadmium and other heavy metals, nitrates, fluoride, chlorine, and trihalomethanes.[52] Over 700 chemicals had been identified in drinking water by 1984. Federal agencies received reports of 34 outbreaks involving disease-tainted drinking water, just between 1991 and 1992. Fifty percent of those cases were the result of the malfunction of purification facilities.[53] Probably the most well known and lethal case in recent years was the 1993 outbreak of cryptosporidium in Milwaukee. Over 400,000 people were sickened and 100 people died before the problem was brought under control.

The latest report from the Environmental Protection Agency found the water systems of 819 cities providing service to 30 million people exceeded the "safe" lead levels established by the Safe Water Drinking Act.[54] The Center for Disease Control and the Environmental Protection Agency have warned that because of increasing outbreaks of cryptosporidium bacteria, cancer patients, organ transplant recipients, and anyone with a weakened immune system should avoid drinking tap water.

The sources of water contaminants are numerous. They include run-off of pesticides from agricultural areas, commercial lawn fertilizers, leaks from improperly stored or dumped toxic waste, landfills, paints, septic tanks used in rural areas, and antiquated sewer systems that fail to properly treat water before releasing it into rivers and lakes. Heavy metals such as cadmium and lead often find their way into the water system from aging galvanized pipes. Nitrates, a known human carcinogen, are usually the result of chemical fertilizer run-off. Even hospitals have been found to dump low-level radioactive waste into the sewers.[55]

Fluoride

There are too many health problems associated with fluoride for us to sit back and hope that, if we put it in our water, it will take care of our teeth. The fact is, evidence shows fluoride toxicity to be "linked with genetic damage in plants and animals, birth defects in humans, especially Down's syndrome, plus a whole series of allergic reactions ranging from fatigue, headaches, urinary tract irritations, diarrhea, and many others."[56]

For years we have accepted as dogma the notion that fluoride in our drinking water helps prevent tooth decay. While there is scientific research supporting the use of fluoride in toothpaste, no scientific research exists to support its use in drinking water. Yet with some of the highest levels of drinking water fluoridation, the United States also has the distinction of having one of the highest levels of tooth decay. In truth, tooth decay is primarily due to the large consumption of sugars in the United States coupled with poor tooth maintenance (i.e., faulty and inconsistent brushing and flossing habits). Furthermore, in areas where the municipal water systems are high in fluoride, children may develop permanent rust-like stains or "mottling" on their teeth.

Chlorine

Chlorine is deliberately placed in our drinking water system as a means of "purifying" it. The reality is quite the contrary. While chlorine does kill some bacteria and other potentially offending matter, studies have linked chlorination with liver, kidney, rectal, and bladder cancers,[57] cancer of the breast, prostate, and testicles, and learning disabilities in children.[58] Recently, a United States-Canadian advisory commission released a statement urging that both countries place an immediate ban on the sale of chlorine because of what it called "startling health problems."[59]

How chlorine harms us is not fully understood, but researchers believe that once in the body, the chemical mimics the hormone estrogen, excesses of which have long been associated with breast cancer in women and reproductive problems in men. There is a double risk with chlorine because of its tendency to interact negatively with other substances. Natural organic matter and other substances, when mixed with chlorine, create a chemical reaction that results in the production of cancer-causing trihalomethanes (THMs) or haloforms, compounds that promote the production of harmful free radicals.[60] (Free radicals will be discussed in detail in Chapter Seven.)

Lead

Lead contamination from drinking water has become a big problem. The most recent EPA survey found 130 municipal water systems exceeding "safe" lead levels and 10 systems with levels that exceeded allowable levels by four times. Excess levels of lead are known to cause damage to the brain, nervous system, kidneys, and red blood cells. Lead has been found to be a particular threat to children and pregnant women since even low levels have been found to cause anemia and damage to children's immune system, low birth weight (a leading cause of infant mortality), learning disabilities, behavioral problems, and retarded growth. Homes and apartment complexes constructed before the 1980s were likely to have had pipes installed that contained lead. After that time, lead regulations forced builders to use lead-free materials.

WATER FILTRATION

All told, the EPA says, "More than 740 million pounds of toxic chemicals pour into waterways annually, in addition to tons of other pollutants ranging from used motor oil to raw sewage."[61] Nobody concerned about their health should be drinking from or bathing in this toxic soup!

Many people have chosen to purchase bottled water to protect themselves against lead and other pollutants. While some brands offer nothing other than partially treated tap water, there are several reputable national brands that print both the source of their water and its chemical nature. Buying bottled water at the supermarket can become expensive, however, and the accumulation of plastic bottles is harmful to the environment. You may prefer a water delivery service. Because water is provided in bulk (usually five-gallon containers), it is less expensive than supermarket liters. Also, these delivery services re-use their delivery bottles, making them more environmentally sound.

Another option is to install a water purification system in your home, allowing you to save on bottles and/or delivery costs, and also protecting the environment. Let's look at a few of the different "point-of-use" filtration systems available to learn which might be your best choice.

Carafe Filter

A carafe filter is clearly the easiest and most inexpensive filter one can use. As the name implies, this system is composed of a carafe with two internal compartments. Water is poured into the top compartment and slowly trickles through the filter and into the lower compartment. While such a system may cost only $25–$35, it has a maximum capacity of one gallon and requires 20 minutes to purify. Unfortunately, carafe systems do not typically perform well in reducing lead. If lead is a problem in your system, this is one filter that won't be helpful.

Activated Carbon

An activated carbon system effectively removes chlorine, herbicides, lead, hydrogen sulfide, and other organic chemicals. This filter uses carbon, which attracts contaminants like a magnet. Filters can range in cost from $40 to $200 for countertop models. Whole-house systems that cover all taps, showers, tubs, and ice makers run between $500 and $1,000.

Solid-Carbon Filtration

Solid carbon filtration effectively removes bad tastes and odors, chlorine, THMs, asbestos, lead, and most pesticides, as well as giardia and cryptosporidium. Small units can be mounted to faucet heads for as little as $25. Countertop systems begin at $225. Whole-house systems can be purchased for between $400 and $800. A word of caution: carbon filters should be replaced according to the manufacturer's recommendation. Carbon filters that are not changed promptly can easily breed harmful bacteria.

Distillation

Distillation will effectively remove arsenic, cadmium, chromium, iron, lead, giardia cysts, nitrates, and sulfates. In this system water is brought to a boiling point. The purified water is turned to vapor, then condensed to a liquid again and stored in a holding container. Since lead's boiling point is higher than water's, the lead is left out. Systems cost between $200–$900 for countertop models and $800–$4,000 for whole-house systems. The disadvantages of a distiller system are that it requires electricity to operate and it removes most of the beneficial minerals in water, making the water nutritionally inferior and poor tasting. Also, distillation is extremely slow, requiring up to seven hours to purify a gallon of water. If your water needs are high, it probably is not the right choice.

Reverse Osmosis

Reverse osmosis (R.O.) removes all minerals and most contaminants with the exception of chlorine and some bacteria. Although this system is wasteful, using three to six gallons of water to produce one gallon of purified water, it is by far the most thorough. Reverse osmosis should be your choice if your drinking water supply contains high levels of lead. An R.O. system is the most effective means to filter lead, removing 98–99 percent in most cases. Some systems combine a reverse osmosis filter system with an activated carbon "post-filter" that acts to catch any remaining organic chemicals that pass by the R.O. filter. This combination is hard to beat. Models range in price from $399 to $1,500. *Note:* R.O. systems are fairly complex to install and will likely require professional assistance.

Other Purchasing Considerations

Currently, there are over 20 major brands of water filters offered on the market. While the most important factor to consider is the degree to which a filter purifies water, there are a few other considerations.

1. How does the unit actually perform?

Some filters are nothing other than taste and odor units and do little to protect your health. While an eager salesperson can provide some very convincing "facts," the best way to confirm filter performance is to ask for a "performance data sheet." Also, while most filters may provide lead filtration, the degree to which lead is removed will vary. The performance data sheet will list how well the filter stands up to a variety of the most harmful substances found in drinking water, as well as inform you whether it has been certified by your State Department of Health Services and other third-party organizations such as the highly respected National Sanitation Foundation (NSF).

2. What is the "service cycle" of the unit?

In other words, how often will you need to replace the filter? While some filter systems have filters that need to be replaced after 250 gallons, others can go for a full 500 gallons before they are in need of replacement. The cost of the replacement filters is another consideration.

3. What is the "flow rate" of the unit?

Some units, while filtering well, may provide only a "dribble" of purified water at a time. Flow rate is stated in "gallons per minute," and can make quite a difference, particularly for family use.

4. Does the unit have a customer satisfaction guarantee and warranty?

If all other factors are equal, a guarantee and warranty can make an important difference to many customers.

THE MICRONUTRIENTS

One must eat to live, not live to eat.
– Molière

VITAMINS AND MINERALS

Vitamins are organic substances that are indispensable in the regulation of chemical reactions in the body, including the conversion of food into energy (metabolism), growth, and development. Although some of the flashy packaging of vitamin supplements might lead you to believe otherwise, vitamins do not provide energy and are neither "revitalizers" nor miracle pills. While a number of the B-complex vitamins act as coenzymes in the production of energy, by themselves they are not an energy source. There is, however, plentiful scientific evidence to confirm that vitamins play a crucial role in both the prevention and treatment of certain diseases and imbalances in the human body. In their absence, a multitude of important processes can be disturbed.

Vitamins can be divided into two groups: fat-soluble and water-soluble. The fat-soluble type (A, D, E, and K) are stored in the body and can become toxic in excessive amounts. The water-soluble variety (B_1, B_2, B_6, B_{12}, and C), are not stored in the body, and excesses are simply excreted in the urine.

Minerals are inorganic (not of plant or animal origin) compounds that primarily make up the "hard" portions of the body such as nails, teeth, and bones. Minerals are responsible for a myriad of processes including the maintenance of blood volume and nerve tissue, cellular water balance, and muscular contraction.

ANTIOXIDANTS

Lately the media has devoted enormous attention to the role of certain vitamins believed to combat free-radical production. These vitamins are known as antioxidants.

Scientists have long understood the danger of free-radical production in the body, but have only recently embraced the concept that nutrition may have a profound influence on it.

Oxidation, a normal metabolic process in the body, occurs when molecules either lose electrons or gain oxygen. In the process, some molecules become highly unstable and can damage other molecules nearby. These highly reactive molecules are called free radicals, and, unchecked, they can convert non-radical molecules into free radicals. Free radicals can also penetrate the cellular membrane and damage the DNA of adjoining cells, creating what are known as oxidative lesions. Unabated, this process can continue as a chain reaction of destruction.

The production of free radicals and DNA lesions is happening continuously in many tissues of the body, including the heart, skin, eyes, and lungs – even the DNA of sperm are under attack.

If this is a normal metabolic process, why aren't we all overwhelmed by free-radical production and cancerous cells? The reason is that our cells have a strong line of defense against this process; they are known as antioxidants.

While there are dozens of antioxidants, the three that are best understood include beta carotene (the plant form of vitamin A), vitamin C and vitamin E. These antioxidants work by allowing themselves to become oxidized instead of the cells.

Evidence confirms that the oxidation process plays a key role in the degeneration of the arterial walls (atherogenesis), and thus the development of atherosclerosis and heart disease, lung disease, cancer, cataracts, immune system dysfunction and even Parkinson's disease, as well as a general acceleration of the aging process.[62] Studies show that coronary heart disease is often associated with low levels of vitamins C, E, and beta carotene.[63] Researchers have concluded that cataracts are caused by oxidation of eye cells by ultraviolet light from the sun. Cataracts, a clouding of the eyes, are a major health problem in the United States. Surgery to remove cataracts is one of the most common operations performed, and comes with an annual price tag of over $3 billion. Based upon studies in which subjects were administered daily supplements, it is estimated that in those who maintain high blood levels of vitamins C and E, the risk for the disease is lowered to one-third.[64] It also appears that T-cells, B-cells, and NK cells, which form the core of the immune system, become impaired by oxidation. Consequently, the body's defense against bacteria, viruses, and even tumor cells is compromised measurably. In a recent double-blind study (i.e., neither the researchers nor the volunteers knew who was receiving additional supplementation) reported in the *American Journal of Clinical Nutrition*, nutritionist Simin Meydani found that those volunteers whose diet was supplemented with 800 I.U. of vitamin E enjoyed a "significant increase in their immune response when compared to an un-supplemented group" (which received only 15 I.U. of vitamin E).[65] Vitamin E has also been found to be essential in protecting the lungs from damage. Not only does it provide protection to the various tissues of the body, but it also acts as an antioxidant for another antioxidant – beta carotene.

Oxidative lesions to sperm DNA have been found to increase up to 250 percent when there are insufficient levels of the antioxidant vitamin C. This, in turn, increases the risk of birth defects and childhood cancer in offspring.

As mentioned before, normal metabolism results in oxidation of cells. However, there are a number of external factors that act as oxidants as well. They include sunlight, cigarette smoke, X rays, food additives, and iron.

OXIDANTS

Sunlight

Sunlight is an oxidative risk factor for skin cells. Beta carotene, a pro-vitamin or precursor of vitamin A, works with the skin cells, protecting them from degeneration and possibly cancer as a consequence of sun exposure. Those who have adequate intakes of beta carotene have an added protection from the harsh rays of the sun.

Cigarette Smoke

Oxides in the nitrogen contained in cigarette smoke not only deplete levels of antioxidants, but also oxidize fat, which can lead to heart disease. Even second-hand smoke has been shown to deplete vitamin C stores in those who are exposed to it. To maintain adequate protection, it is estimated that cigarette smokers must consume between two and three times the amount of vitamin C as non-smokers. Cigarette smoke also disables vitamin E, thwarting its ability to effectively protect the lungs. Studies in both the United States and Europe have shown consistently that the risk for lung cancer is reduced when levels of beta carotene are kept high.[66]

Food Additives

Certain processed food additives have also been earmarked as participants in oxidation. For instance, nitrates, which are commonly used to preserve smoked and cured meats such as bacon, act as oxidants when they are ingested. This is because, inside the intestine, nitrates combine with amino acids and form substances called nitrosamines, which are known to cause cancer.[67]

Iron

We have always been told that it is important to get plenty of iron in our diet. The problem is that few people understand which foods are good sources of iron, and that an excess of iron may be dangerous. Although iron can be found in meat and other animal products (called hem-iron), this type of iron has been found to facilitate the production of free radicals. Those whose diets are centered around meat have a very high intake of this type of iron. Unlike water-soluble vitamins, whose excesses are excreted from the body, iron excesses accumulate in the body. In fact, some Americans have a genetic predisposition to hemochromatosis, a condition in which iron accumulation in the body reaches toxic levels. Some experts have estimated that the average man may be holding onto 1,000–2,000 mg of needless iron which may facilitate free radical production and contribute to the destruction of cells. In addition, because iron oxidizes cholesterol, its presence further increases the risk of developing heart disease. A recent study of nearly 2,000 Finnish men found that those who had higher stores of iron in their body were more likely to suffer a heart attack.

IRON CONTENT OF VARIOUS FOODS (mg per 1 cup)	
SPINACH	6.4 mg
PINTO BEANS	5.4 mg
WHOLE-WHEAT FLOUR	5.2 mg
CHICKPEAS	4.9 mg
SOYBEANS	4.9 mg
BARLEY	4.2 mg
LENTILS	4.2 mg
PEAS	3.4 mg
PUMPKIN	3.4 mg
RAISINS	3.0 mg

Most recently, research is pointing at excessive iron stores as a major contributor to the development of Parkinson's disease.[68] It has been found that iron accumulates in a specific region of the brain known as the substantia nigra where the dopamine neurons are concentrated and vulnerable to damage. Researchers are now looking into antioxidant therapies for those who may be prone to this disease.

All of this is not to say that one should avoid iron. Iron is essential to the formation of blood cells, the transportation of oxygen, and the maintenance of tissues. Fortunately, there is plenty of iron available in a vegetarian diet. Like the protein found in plant foods, iron is supplied in plants in moderate amounts. Further, the form of iron found in plant foods is absorbed more conservatively by the body. For these reasons, the chances of consuming excesses of iron and building up dangerous stores in the body are minimized.

You may be relieved to know that in studies of vegetarians who follow a balanced diet similar to the Revised American Diet, all individuals were found to have adequate intakes of iron.[69]

ANTIOXIDANT-RICH FOODS

It is perfectly clear that when the body is deficient in antioxidants, we increase our chances of developing diseases and illness. Therefore, we should strive to maintain a "stockpile" of antioxidants, which are found in abundance in fruits and vegetables. The more fruit-and-vegetable-rich your diet is, the better prepared your body will be to defend you from free-radical production. Dr. Bruce Ames, Professor of Biochemistry and Molecular Biology at the University of California, Berkeley, and a leader in the field of cancer research, states "The incidence of most types of cancer is double among people who eat few fruits and vegetables as compared to those who eat about five portions per day." By following the fruit-and-vegetable-rich diet outlined in this book, you cannot help but meet, if not exceed, that suggested quota. On the other hand, animal products such as meat, fish, and milk contain an array of pesticides, antibiotics, hormones, and other chemical residues which only heighten the risk of disease. So each time animal foods are consumed, they displace other antioxidant-rich foods and the risk for disease escalates.

Now that the importance of antioxidants has been established, let's look at the best sources for them.

As far as beta carotene goes, carrots and sweet potatoes are the champs. One cup contains 12 and 15 mg of beta carotene, respectively. Most people know that an orange is rich in vitamin C – a medium orange contains about 80 mg – yet few people know that a cup of sweet red peppers contains a whopping 190 mg of vitamin C! For vitamin E sources, look to corn, chickpeas, sweet potatoes, wheat germ, soybeans, whole grains, and vegetables. In general, beta carotene is found in yellow and green vegetables, leafy greens, and fruits, while vitamin C is found in citrus fruits, strawberries, and green vegetables.

FOOD	FOODS RICH IN ANTIOXIDANTS		
	VITAMIN C (MG)	BETA CAROTENE (MG)	VITAMIN E (MG)
BROCCOLI 1/2 CUP	49	0.7	0.9
CANTALOUPE 1 CUP	68	3.1	0.3
CARROT 1 MED	7	12.2	0.3
KALE 1/2 CUP	27	2.9	3.7
MANGO 1 MED	57	4.8	2.3
PUMPKIN 1/2 CUP	5	10.5	1.1
RED PEPPER 1/2 CUP	95	1.7	0.3
SPINACH 1/2 CUP	9	4.4	2.0
STRAWBERRIES 1 CUP	86	0	0.3
SWEET POTATO 1 MED	28	14.9	5.5

VITAMIN SUPPLEMENTATION

There is an ongoing and heated debate about whether the average person needs to take vitamin and mineral supplements. The FDA asserts that anyone should be able to obtain the necessary vitamins and minerals through a well-balanced diet. This is true. The question is, how many people are consuming a well-balanced diet? Very few. According to the National Center for Health Statistics, only 9 percent of

MINERALS AND THEIR SOURCES

	U.S.R.D.A	VEGAN SOURCES	DEFICIENCY SYMPTOMS	FUNCTIONS	DEPLETES/ INHIBITS
Calcium	800 mg 1,200 mg (preg/lact.)	Leafy green vegetables, broccoli, collard, kale, almonds, tofu, fortified soy products	Brittle bones, heart palpitations, muscle pain, tooth decay	Required for development and maintenance of bones and teeth. Important to blood clotting, nerve transmission, heart rhythm, and contraction and expansion of muscles.	Excess protein, caffeine, magnesium deficiency
Chromium	None established	Whole-grain cereals, corn oil, brown rice potatoes, brewer's yeast	Retarded growth, atherosclerosis	Enhances insulin function; stimulates enzymes in metabolism of energy; important in synthesis of fatty acids, cholesterol, and protein.	None
Cobalt	None established	Leafy greens vegetables, fruits	Retarded growth, pernicious anemia	Maintains red blood cells; functions with vitamin B_{12}; activates some enzymes.	None
Copper	2 mg	Soybeans, raisins, nuts, legumes, molasses, avocados, raisins, oats	Skin sores, impaired respiration, general weakness	Important in function of enzymes; with vitamin C it forms elastin; formation of red blood cells; hair and skin; bone formation.	Excessive levels of zinc
Iodine	150 mg	Mushrooms, iodized salt, kelp, onion, garlic, spinach, carrots	Irritability, dry hair, nervous dysfunction, cold hands and feet	Regulates energy production and rate of metabolism; prevents goiter; promotes healthy hair, skin, nails.	None
Iron	10 mg (males) 15 mg (females)	Cherry juice, molasses, wheat germ, leafy green vegetables, shredded wheat, dried fruits, legumes	General weakness, anemia, constipation	Important to formation of hemoglobin and myoglobin; promotes protein metabolism; promotes growth.	Excessive levels of zinc
Magnesium	350 mg (males) 280 mg (females) 350 mg (preg/lact)	Molasses, whole grains, nuts, kelp, bran, green vegetables, seeds, oats	Muscular excitability, nervousness, tremors	Catalyst in the utilization of protein, fats and carbohydrates, phosphorus, calcium. Assists in maintenance of arteries, heart, and nerves.	None
Manganese	None established	Whole grains, nuts, legumes, leafy greens, bananas, celery, pineapple, bran	Hearing loss, dizziness	Enzyme activator; maintains sex hormone production, tissue respiration, skeletal development.	Excessive intakes of phosphorus and calcium
Phosphorus	800 mg 1,200 mg (preg/lact)	Legumes, nuts, whole grains; sesame, sunflower, and pumpkin seeds; garlic	Weight loss, appetite suppression, fatigue, nervousness	Works with calcium to maintain bones, teeth; cell growth and repair; heart muscle contraction; nerve activity.	Excessive intakes of magnesium, aluminum, and iron
Potassium	None established	Whole grains, legumes, sunflower seeds, dried fruit, peaches, nuts, molasses, bananas	Respiratory dysfunction, poor reflexes, dry skin, nervousness, irregular heartbeat	Controls activity of heart muscle, nervous system, and kidneys; growth; muscle contractions.	Coffee, diuretics, alcohol, cortisone, laxatives
Selenium	None estabished	Broccoli, onions, bran, wheat germ, tomatoes, brown rice, brewer's yeast, whole grains	Premature aging	Beneficial for kwashiorkor; works with vitamin E; preserves tissue elasticity.	None
Zinc	15 mg (males) 12 mg (females)	Soybeans, brewer's yeast, spinach, legumes, mushrooms, sunflower and pumpkin seeds	Delayed sexual maturity, inhibition of taste, suppressed appetite, fatigue, retarded growth	Assists in digestion and metabolism of protein, carbohydrates and phosphorus; component of insulin; prostate gland function.	Phosphorus deficiency, alcohol

CHAPTER EIGHT

THE REVISED AMERICAN DIET ™

You will observe with concern how long a useful truth may be known and exist,
before it is generally received and practiced on.
– Benjamin Franklin

So far, we have seen how influential diet is for good health. Clearly, through good nutrition, all of us can easily and dramatically enhance our well-being. Some of us may be in grave danger because of our dietary habits; yet each of us has the choice to take control and create effective change. I want to stress that what I am proposing is not another fad diet, but a comprehensive change in the type and quantity of foods you consume. In the following pages you will find guidelines and suggestions for following the Revised American Diet. With this diet, you will reap many rewards – rewards that will last a lifetime.

We have already looked at some of the abundant scientific evidence indicating humans will benefit greatly by following a diet that excludes animal products. Let's look more closely to see why.

The current national guidelines suggest a cholesterol intake of no more than 300 mg a day. If Americans actually ate anywhere near this amount, you would not see anyone consuming eggs at your local breakfast house. This is because a single egg nearly meets the entire current, daily recommendation for cholesterol intake. The Revised American Diet doesn't recommend any cholesterol intake, because the body has no need for an external source of cholesterol; as I mentioned earlier, it produces all the cholesterol it needs internally. The reality is that the less cholesterol we take in through diet, the lower our risk for disease. From a health standpoint, the ideal choice is to consume no cholesterol at all. The only way to achieve a zero-cholesterol diet is to consume no animal products, as only animal foods contain cholesterol.

When you make the transition from a diet that is centered on high-fat animal products to a diet centered on whole grains, vegetables, legumes, and fruits, you need not be concerned with percentages and grams per serving calculations because the recommended foods are significantly lower in fat, have moderate levels of protein, and contain no cholesterol. They are also naturally high in complex carbohydrates. Whole grains, vegetables, legumes, and fruits are all "nutrient-dense," meaning they naturally contain higher levels of the micronutrients (vitamins and minerals), important phytochemicals, and beneficial fiber our body needs. The types of food you choose to eat – not the exact measurement of such foods – make a desirable nutrient balance possible. Weighing foods, counting calories, and calculating fat grams per serving becomes a thing of the past.

BENEFITS OF THE RAD

You may be asking yourself by now, "Okay, so this is a healthier way of eating, but what exactly will I gain from following such a diet?" You have already seen the many diseases that are likely to develop as a consequence of following the Standard American Diet. By following the RAD, you will gain significant protection from those diseases. In addition, there are several additional benefits that you can expect.

1. Increased energy

Who couldn't use more energy throughout the day? Invariably, people who make the transition to a diet low in fat and high in complex carbohydrates find they have increased energy. There are a couple of reasons for this. First, because of their high fat content, heavy meats, eggs, and dairy products require a longer time to be broken down and assimilated by the body. Digestion requires energy diverted from other bodily needs. Consequently, we feel slow and lethargic. Moreover, high-fat animal-source foods, contrary to popular belief, are poor sources of energy. In fact, they are very low in complex carbohydrates. Complex carbohydrates are the best source of lasting energy for the body. The whole-grain products, vegetables, and legumes that replace these high-fat foods are all rich in complex carbohydrates. For an example, look at the following chart.

| FOOD | CARBOHYDRATE COMPARISON | |
	Serving	Carbohydrates
BAKED POTATO	3 $^1/_2$ oz.	25 grams
Pork Loin		0 grams
PINTO BEANS	3 $^1/_2$ oz.	26 grams
Chicken Breast		0 grams
WHOLE-WHEAT SPAGHETTI	3 $^1/_2$ oz.	28 grams
Cheddar Cheese		1 gram
DATES	3 $^1/_2$ oz.	74 grams
Milk		5 grams

2. Easy and permanent weight loss

The FDA currently lists nearly 30,000 diets. At any one time, it is estimated that 65 million Americans are on some form of weight-loss diet, whether it be one promoted in a fashion magazine or at one of the thousands of weight-loss centers around the country. This is a clear indication of how confused and unsuccessful people are when it comes to controlling their body weight. If any of these diets worked and was a healthy and safe way of eating, there would be no market for the other 29,999 diets. Some diets, such as liquid protein, are life-threatening, resulting in heart arrhythmia and, in some cases, death.

Many fad diets that prescribe extremely low-calorie and/or carbohydrate intake do see rapid weight loss. However, the loss is generally in lean body mass (muscle and water), as well as in glycogen stores. Unfortunately, many people will misinterpret this as a fat loss when they step on their scale. In 95 percent of cases, after a restrictive fad diet, the body regains the lost weight. What is worse is that the weight is regained not in the form it was lost (muscle and water), but as fat instead! Do you know any chronic dieters? If so, you have probably heard them tell you that they suddenly stop losing weight on their diets, eventually gain it all back and feel even worse. Here is why.

Most conventional fad diets prescribe a highly restrictive calorie intake. When an individual drops his or her calorie consumption significantly, the body moves to a state of alert. No, you won't hear bells and whistles going off, but inside changes are occurring. In fact, the body interprets this reduction in calories as potential starvation. If starvation is "just around the corner," what do you think your body will do to prepare? That's right, conserve! The body shifts into "survival mode" and begins to slow the metabolism, burning fewer calories (up to 15 percent less) and holding on to fat reserves as a way of assuring itself a lasting supply of energy. Essentially, it operates with less. This is why dieters say, "At first the weight dropped off like magic, then suddenly I couldn't lose a pound." While this safety mechanism is a wonderful response to actual starvation, it is extremely frustrating for someone attempting to lose weight. Even though fat cells may shrink to a degree (the number of fat cells stays the same), they are very sensitized and "anxious" to gain back what they lost after a short-term diet ends. In fact, research has shown that with each successive diet a chronic dieter follows, not only does she regain more weight more easily, but her metabolic rate continues to slow further each time. Furthermore, people who are on calorie-restricted diets don't feel well. They feel deprived of food, lack energy, and become irritable.

What is the solution to this madness? Simply, reduce your fat intake, not your calorie intake. Our bodies are highly complex organisms that are conducting thousands of processes an hour. To carry out all these tasks – not to mention fuel our daily activities – energy is required, and energy comes from food. Massive cutbacks in calories mean massive cutbacks in energy and dysfunction all around the table. When you eat a diet that is low in fat, rich in whole grains, and high in fiber, it is not another temporary diet. It is not something you begin a few weeks before the senior prom, before a day at the beach, or in order to fit into a particular outfit. It is a way of life, a comprehensive change from the SAD.

FOOD	FAT COMPARISON	
	Serving	Fat
BANANA	3 $^1/_2$ oz.	1 gram
Ground Beef		21 grams
BROWN RICE	3 $^1/_2$ oz.	1 gram
Roasted Ham		21 grams
BAKED POTATO	3 $^1/_2$ oz.	0 grams
Cheddar Cheese		33 grams
OATMEAL	3 $^1/_2$ oz.	1 gram
Pepperoni		39 grams

Much of the struggle with weight many people experience is the result of the types of food they eat, not the quantity. To illustrate, each gram of fat yields nine calories, while a gram of either carbohydrate or protein has only four. Consequently, on a traditional high-fat diet, you consume excessive amounts of calories before achieving a feeling of satiety, and before satisfying the body's nutritional needs. On the RAD, however, when eating primarily whole grains, vegetables, and fruits, you can actually eat more, without gaining weight. Again, we can look to China as a model. The Chinese consume 20 percent more calories than Americans, yet Americans are about 25 percent fatter. Why? Only 15 percent of their calories come from fat – fat that is primarily derived from plant sources. Plainly put, people who follow a vegetarian diet are consistently slimmer than those who consume a diet centered on animal products.

You simply cannot feel deprived of food on a low-fat diet. You would need to consume over 15 cups of brown rice before you would take in as much fat as in a single cup of whole milk, and over 50 cups of broccoli before equaling the amount of fat in a cheeseburger. Imagine eating fifty bananas. Impossible, right? Yet that's what you would have to do in order to get the same amount of fat in an average 12-oz. steak. Look at the previous chart that compares the fat content of animal and plant foods.

3.   Controlled insulin production

Insulin is a hormone produced by the pancreas and released in the body to help balance blood sugar. The greater the amount of sugar released in the blood, the more insulin is necessary to remove the sugar and transport it to waiting cells. Unfortunately, once blood sugar levels drop, two things happen: energy levels are lowered so one feels tired, and appetite increases. With an increase in appetite comes an increase in eating. So, it makes sense that to help control our appetite and maintain a more stable supply of energy, we maintain lower levels of insulin.

The refined carbohydrates and high-fat foods found in the Standard American Diet lead to increased insulin production. This is one reason why the average American can never seem to get enough food. When he ingests refined foods such as white flour, sugar, and many sweets, the sugar content enters his blood very rapidly, raising blood sugar levels too fast. The opposite effect occurs when he eats whole, unrefined foods found in the Revised American Diet. These foods are largely complex carbohydrates and contain significant amounts of fiber. They are assimilated by the body more gradually than refined foods. For this reason, less insulin production is required, and a roller-coaster appetite is avoided.

Depending on the level of body fat one begins with, people who are overweight and follow the Revised American Diet, in conjunction with the other components of Whole Health Living, usually lose about 10 – 15 pounds a month. Once their body approaches a comfortable and healthy weight, the loss begins to taper off. The difference is that when they adopt the principles of the RAD, the weight stays off permanently!

4. Lowered blood pressure

Although the human body can function on 500–1,000 mg of sodium daily, in reality the Standard American Diet contains somewhere between 3,000 and 6,000 mg a day. In addition to the many other factors mentioned, an excess of sodium plays an important role in high blood pressure. Chinese physicians knew this as far back as 4,500 years ago when they said, "Hence if too much salt is used in food, the pulse hardens."[71] It works like this: when the body is overwhelmed with sodium, it begins to retain water. Consequently, the volume of blood being transported in the body increases. The blood vessels automatically compensate by contracting, thereby reducing blood flow. However, this compounds the problem, as the heart is required to work even harder to move the blood through the narrowed blood vessels.

The Revised American Diet is naturally low in sodium. In the following charts, the first one shows the difference in sodium levels between animal-food and plant-food sources, and the second indicates sources of hidden sodium, typically found in prepackaged foods.

FOOD	SODIUM COMPARISON	
	Serving	Sodium
STRAWBERRIES	1 cup	1 mg
Ham	3 oz.	1,203 mg
ZUCCHINI	1 cup	3 mg
Hot Dog	4 oz.	1,146 mg
BROCCOLI	1 cup	17 mg
Blue Cheese	1 cup	1,884 mg
BROWN RICE	1 cup	5 mg
Sausage	3 oz.	890 mg

	OTHER SOURCES OF SODIUM
BAKING POWDER	Baked goods.
BAKING SODA (SODIUM BICARBONATE)	Baked goods, an alkalizer for indigestion.
DISODIUM PHOSPHATE	Quick-cooking cereals, processed cheese.
MONOSODIUM GLUTAMATE (MSG)	Seasoning used in restaurants, (particularly Chinese), packaged, canned, and frozen foods. Commercially available in product called Accent.
SALT (SODIUM CHLORIDE)	Canned, frozen and preserved foods. Used at the table for taste.
SODIUM ALGINATE	Chocolate milk and ice cream for smooth texture.
SODIUM BENZOATE	A preservative in ketchup, mustard, relish and salad dressings.
SODIUM HYDROXIDE	Olives, fruits and vegetables.
SODIUM NITRATE	Packaged meats and sausages.
SODIUM PROPIONATE	Preservative in pasteurized cheese, cakes, and breads.
SODIUM SULFITE	A bleach on artificially colored fruits and a preservative of dried fruits.
PRESCRIPTION/OVER-THE-COUNTER DRUGS; IBUPROFEN	Many prescription and over-the-counter drugs contain sodium. To be sure, ask your physician.

5.   Lowered blood cholesterol

An elevated cholesterol level is a strong predictor of heart disease and stroke. On a conventional high-cholesterol diet, we run about a 50 percent chance of suffering a heart attack sometime in our life. That's like playing Russian Roulette! When you eliminate animal products from your diet, however, you eliminate all sources of cholesterol and your blood cholesterol level will drop significantly. Look at the following chart to see the level of cholesterol in various animal foods. (*Note:* One egg nearly equals the maximum suggested daily intake for cholesterol [300 mg] on the Standard American Diet.)

FOOD	CHOLESTEROL COMPARISON	
	Serving	Mg
ALL GRAINS	1	0 mg
Egg		275 mg
ALL VEGETABLES	3 $^1/_2$ oz	0 mg
Goose		96 mg
ALL FRUITS	3 $^1/_2$ oz	0 mg
Sour Cream		116 mg
ALL LEGUMES	3 $^1/_2$ oz	0 mg
Chicken Breast		85 mg

6.   Reduced intake of hormones, pesticides, and antibiotics

Farm animals are commonly treated with growth-inducing hormones and disease-preventing antibiotics, and eat feed that often contains pesticide residues. Some experts believe that residues of pesticides, as well as the hormones commonly found in meat, contribute to escalating cancer rates in humans. So serious has the hormone problem become in the United States, that the European Economic Community (EEC) has now placed a ban on the importation of any hormone-treated meat from the United States.[72] Large amounts of antibiotics are routinely fed to cattle to keep them from getting sick. None of us needs more antibiotics in our bodies, and some people are highly allergic to them. While you may not recognize the names, chloramphenicol, cabadox, nitrofurazone, dimetridazole, and ipronidazole are all chemicals, the residues of which have been detected in the United States' meat supply.[73] Many of these chemicals are known human carcinogens. You'll never need to worry about vegetables, fruits, legumes, and grains containing hormones and antibiotics.

CHAPTER NINE

FOODS TO ELIMINATE

We are not carnivores and never have been carnivores,
and that should be remembered.
—Dr. Richard Leakey, Paleoanthropologist

MEAT

I have memories as a child of chewing endlessly on a piece of meat until my jaws became tired. At that point, I would simply swallow the piece and hope it fit down my throat. It always bothered me that I had to work so hard to consume meat. Adults told me that I simply didn't chew long enough – that eating meat properly required that one chew each piece at least 35 times. For years I continued to eat meat, sometimes counting in my head, other times forgetting and just swallowing (uneasily) a chunk of meat.

It was not until many years later that I discovered why all that chewing was required. If one looks at the evolutionary history of human beings, we have primarily been herbivores, or plant eaters, until relatively recently. In support of this fact, our teeth are mostly flat for grinding plant foods, unlike the teeth of carnivores, or meat eaters, which are pointed and sharp, designed for effectively piercing and tearing flesh. Even our clawless hands are useless for this purpose. Moreover, I learned that carnivores also have the capacity to assimilate, process, and rid themselves of the massive amounts of cholesterol they consume on a daily basis. Consequently, they do not suffer from atherosclerosis or "hardening of the arteries." The human liver, on the other hand, has only a limited capacity to contend with large amounts of dietary cholesterol and, consequently, excesses lead to disease.

Even our intestinal tract is different from that of carnivores. Other herbivores, like humans, have long intestinal tracts that are suited for digesting plant foods. Carnivores, on the other hand, have very short tracts best suited for the digestion of meat. However, even with these clear physiological differences, we humans manage to eat meat, even if we have to chew 20, 30, or 40 times or more, and we pay a heavy price for it.

As we have seen so far, meat is one of the primary sources of saturated fat and cholesterol in the American diet and, therefore, is a major influence in the development of many diseases. We also have learned that meat contains excessive levels of iron, which acts as an oxidant, leading to the production of free radicals. Free radicals not only cause cellular damage and expedite the aging process of tissues, but also are linked to cancer and birth defects. Another major drawback of meat consumption is that meat is totally lacking in fiber, which is very important in controlling weight, preventing colon cancer, and stimulating immune function.

Women who eat meat once a day
have a breast cancer risk 380 percent higher
than women who eat meat once a week.[74]

As we discussed previously, meat is also often tainted with chemical pesticides, fertilizers, and hormone residues, many of which have been shown to be carcinogenic to humans. In addition to the hormones with which beef cattle are treated to increase their size rapidly, the meat is often poisoned by the cow's internal hormones (such as adrenaline), which are released during the slaughter of the animals. Livestock are also fed enormous quantities of antibiotic drugs, residues of which remain in the meat for the consumer.

As if these were not sufficient reasons to exclude meat from your diet, there is also the problem of an increasing incidence of bacteria poisoning with meat consumption. E-coli 0157:H7 (commonly referred to as E-coli) is an extremely virulent strain of bacteria that can cause severe illness and even death when present in very small amounts. Paul Cieslak of the Center for Disease Control and Prevention confirms that rates for E-coli poisoning continue to climb. In January 1993 there were over 500 cases reported in Washington state alone. Death resulted in four of the cases involving children. All of these cases were linked to a well-known chain of fast-food restaurants. Several months later, five people in Oregon were hospitalized for having eaten meat tainted with E-coli bacteria. Currently, the Center for Disease Control estimates that there are over 20,000 cases of E-coli poisoning each year.

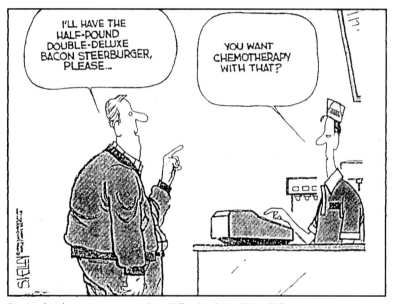

Reprinted with permission courtesy Steve Kelley, San Diego Union Tribune.

Once the bacteria enters the body, it begins damaging the intestinal lining as well as the kidneys. Usually it results in bloody diarrhea. E-coli resides in the intestines and, therefore, the feces of animals. It is during the slaughtering process that the meat inevitably becomes contaminated by this deadly bacteria. Many question why, when the slaughtering procedure has changed little over the past few decades, E-coli has suddenly become such a great threat. In her monumental

Whole Health

book *The Coming Plague*, health and science writer Laurie Garrett demonstrates that it is the unregulated use of large quantities of antibiotics in the raising of livestock that has resulted in a more powerful "mutant strain" of the bacteria.

To reduce the risk of E-coli poisoning, consumers are told to enjoy their meat well-cooked. Ironically though, the longer meat is cooked, the more it develops Heterocyclic Amines, a cancer-causing agent that forms when animal protein is heated excessively. In fact, according to a recent National Cancer Institute study, those who eat their meat medium-well to well-done are three times more likely to develop stomach cancer than those who eat meat rare. Meat that is "charred," as often occurs in barbecuing, develops another class of carcinogens known as Polycyclic Aromatic hydrocarbons.[75]

CHICKEN

As the health risks associated with red meat have become better known and its consumption continues to decline, many people have turned to poultry as a lower-fat alternative. Granted, poultry does usually contain a bit less fat than red meat, but it is still saturated fat. Yet ounce for ounce it contains the same amount of cholesterol as beef. Furthermore, as with meat, there are certain risks associated with eating chicken, aside from its saturated fat and cholesterol content. The biggest concern is over bacterial contamination, a problem that has become quite serious. According to the Center for Disease Control, each year nearly 2,000 Americans die from such bacterial poisoning.[76] The number of people who get sick from eating chicken each year has risen to 6.5 million.[77] The most common forms of bacteria include Salmonella and Campylobacter, and the latest estimates are that at least 60 percent of chickens in the United States are contaminated with these and other microorganisms.

Much has been written about the unsanitary conditions in which animals are processed and how these conditions increase the chances of contamination. While the USDA, under fire by consumer advocates for failing to provide better monitoring and inspection, insists it has cracked down on chicken processors, a recent random sampling of chickens from supermarkets across the country suggests that there still exists considerable risk. In this sampling, 30 different chickens were tested including national brands, non-brands, kosher, and "free-range" varieties. Twenty-one of the chickens were contaminated with Campylobacter, twelve with Lysteria, and eight with Salmonella.

FISH

Fish has also become popular in recent years as a replacement for meat. Yet many of the popular fish, such as salmon and swordfish, are similar in fat content to poultry and meat. For instance, 52 percent of the calories in salmon come from fat. Like the meat it often replaces, fish also contains plenty of cholesterol.

Another increasing problem with fish is their level of contamination. PCBs, DDT, dioxin, mercury, and viruses are detected all too often. Unfortunately, many of the world's oceans have become great big rugs, under which tremendous amounts of toxic, industrial waste are being swept. While we cannot easily see this waste, its presence is reflected in the increasing levels of contamination of fish.

Certain populations who depend on fish, including South American coastal villages and the Arctic Inuits, have been found to have exceptionally high concentrations of these contaminants in their bodies. It is well known that PCBs interfere with estrogenic activity and reproduction, as well as suppress immune system function.[78] Current estimates from the Center for Disease Control are that each year there are over 325,000 cases of illness caused by contaminated seafood.

Consumption of some cold-water fish has been promoted on the grounds that they contain Omega-3 fatty acids, which are thought to provide protection against heart disease because they help prevent blood clotting. Unfortunately, because Omega-3 fatty acids in fish are very unstable, they may lead to the production of free radicals. The popular press has failed to point out that vegetables such as spinach and broccoli, as well as some legumes, pumpkin seed oil, and particularly flaxseed oil also are rich sources of the Omega-3s.

damaged pancreas to produce insulin. Studies of one of the proteins in cow's milk, bovine serum albumin (BSA), have indicated that BSA may instigate an auto-immune response that leads to the destruction of the beta cells of the pancreas.

DRUG CONTAMINATION

Like meat, milk carries a risk of exposure to hormones, pesticides, antibiotics and other chemicals that may end up in the milk supply. In 1993 came the publicity regarding the biosynthetic milk hormone called BGH or BST. Dr. Richard Burroughs, a veterinarian who spent half his 13-year career working for the Food and Drug Administration studying the effects of bovine hormone use in cows, says, "The very first data I saw come in showed that it [BGH] increased reproductive and udder infections in cows." These sick cows, with a condition known as mastitis, then must be treated with sulfa drugs and numerous other antibiotics routinely fed to sick dairy cows.[82] The *Wall Street Journal* conducted an independent investigation of the safety of milk, and their study revealed drug residues in 40 percent of the milk samples taken from 10 major American cities. Contrary to what one would hope, public awareness hasn't mitigated the problem. In the Spring 1996 *FDA Journal*, investigators reported finding 16 illegal drug residues in the cows at an Oregon dairy farm, including streptomycin, neomycin, and gentmicin.[83]

Rather than move into uncharted waters, Europe placed a moratorium on BGH until the year 2000. It now seems clear that the wait was well worth it. The most recent study of BGH is published in the *International Journal of Health Services*, and the news is grim. The study, authored by Samuel Epstein, M.D., professor of environmental toxicology at the University of Illinois, Chicago, shows that BGH may well promote breast, colon, and gastrointestinal cancer in humans.

BEST SOURCE OF CALCIUM? THINK AGAIN

With all of the risks associated with dairy products, why would anyone continue to eat them? Most people are drawn to dairy because it is supposed to be a good source of calcium. What people (including many health practitioners) are not aware of is the fact that cow's milk is more likely a contributor to calcium deficiency. This is because cow's milk is very high in phosphorus and protein. Elevated phosphorus levels make calcium assimilation difficult. When excessive protein is ingested, the blood can become too acidic. To buffer this rise in acid the body draws on calcium stored in the bones, a process known as calcium leaching. The greater a person's protein intake, the higher their calcium losses will be, and regardless of how much calcium is consumed either in the diet or through supplements, this calcium leaching will continue unabated unless the protein consumption is reduced.

Protein-induced calcium losses may be one reason Americans are told to consume 800 to 1,200 milligrams of calcium a day. However, government recommendations in both the United Kingdom and Canada call for a more modest 500 milligrams a day. Even the Food and Agriculture Division of the World Health Organization (WHO) recommends a daily calcium intake of as little as 400 mg a day. It should be noted that WHO also recommends a protein intake of 4.5 percent of one's daily calorie intake–far less than the 12 to 15 percent Americans are told to consume.

In parts of the world where protein intake is moderate and largely derived from plant sources, people are perfectly healthy consuming between 400-500 milligrams of calcium a day, derived primarily from vegetables, grains, roots, nuts and seeds. As previously mentioned, the Bantu women of Africa may have as many as 10 children in their lifetime and consume little or no dairy, yet osteoporosis and tooth decomposition are extremely rare in their population.

Anyone who has studied the composition of foods knows that a variety of whole grains, vegetables, nuts and seeds—such as broccoli, turnip greens, carrots, spinach, cauliflower, kale, onions, almonds and filberts—are excellent sources of calcium. The fact is, more calcium will be absorbed by the body from a cup of broccoli than from a cup of milk! Yet little more than common sense is necessary to destroy the myth of dairy as the best source of calcium. Where do the mighty bovines get their calcium? Certainly not from the milk of another animal. They get it from eating greens. Does it make sense that in order to get the calcium we need, nature planned for humans to be nursing from another species? The image helps one see how preposterous the whole dairy mythology is.

EGGS

Eggs are one of the most concentrated sources of cholesterol. One egg can contain up to 275 mg of cholesterol and about 8 grams of fat. Consuming just one egg per day can increase your blood cholesterol level by 12 percent.[84] Since you now understand the risks associated with elevated cholesterol, I am sure you can see that the current recommendation of a cholesterol intake of 300 mg a day is both excessive and ridiculous. Not only that, it is virtually unattainable if one consumes eggs and/or other animal products. Let me illustrate:

Imagine walking into a local breakfast house one morning. Looking around, you see a lot of eggs being eaten. Whether poached, fried, scrambled, or in an omelet, eggs are the most common choice for breakfast. Now consider the eggs in the pancake and waffle batter or the eggs in the muffins, the coffee cake, or coating the French toast. By eating only a single egg for breakfast, an individual has already nearly reached her maximum cholesterol intake for the day. Realistically, we know that most people will have surpassed the suggested 300 mg by the time they finish their breakfast, and since they will have at least two more meals, they will have two more opportunities to consume cholesterol before the day is finished.

Eggs contain virtually no fiber, and, like dairy products, are a common cause of food allergy. Also, eggs are produced under horrific conditions, in which disease poses a great threat to the chickens. Consequently, the animals are often administered antibiotics and other drugs, the residues of which may end up in the eggs.

CHAPTER TEN

FOODS TO INCLUDE

The Chinese make no distinction between food and medicine.
– Lin Yutang

We have seen which foods we need to eliminate from our diet in our pursuit of Whole Health. Let's now look at the healthful foods we should include.

GRAINS

Around the world grains have played an important part in the diet of many societies. For instance, in Central America corn has been a dietary mainstay, while in the Middle East millet is eaten regularly. In North Africa couscous is popular, and in Italy they enjoy polenta. In Asia rice and bulgur wheat are staples, and in Scotland, oats.

Whole grains are a rich source of fiber, vitamins (particularly B and E), and minerals (particularly magnesium, calcium, and iron) and are an excellent source of complex carbohydrates. Unfortunately, the average American eats very little whole-grain foods. Oddly enough, while we are the largest producer of grain in the world, over half our grain production is used for livestock feed.

A major drawback of the grain consumed in America is that it has often been processed in a way that compromises its nutritional quality. Grains are milled to make them easier to eat and enable them to cook faster. Before they are refined, grains are composed of germ, bran, and endosperm. Some grains may also contain an outer "shell," called the hull. During the milling process, however, much of the bran, vitamins, and minerals are lost.

As an example, let's look at flour. All flour begins in a whole form. However, after a process of grinding, rolling, and sifting the grain, the seed is separated. What is retained is the "powdered" endosperm. This endosperm is then bleached (with chemicals such as benzoyl peroxide, or acetone peroxide) and finally becomes the common white flour you find in the supermarket. When whole-wheat flour is made, all components of the seed are retained and recombined after milling. In refined white flours, over 50 percent of the vitamins and nearly 25 percent of the fiber can be lost, leaving you with a fraction of the original nutritional value.

This is why when shopping for breads you should make sure the label says "whole wheat." Without the word "whole," the bread could be made from a mix of refined and whole grains, or colored, processed grains. The word "whole" is your assurance that the product still contains the bran and germ of the grain.

WHY REFINE GRAINS?

Grains are refined for three reasons. First, the process makes some grains easier to eat. Second, it makes the grain cook faster. Finally, when a grain is refined the natural oil content is removed. Food manufacturers prefer not to have the oil present because it reduces the shelf life of the grain. Health-conscious consumers prefer that the oil be present as it is a rich source of vitamin E. To make up for the lost nutrients, food manufacturers will "enrich" processed food with certain vitamins and minerals; yet, as the chart on the next page illustrates, enriched grains will never equal the nutritional quality of whole grains.

Another problem with the enriching process is that the nutrients may be inadvertently washed away. Most enriched grains are "sprayed" with a nutrient-containing formula. However, rinsing of the grain or excessive water used in cooking may wash away these nutrients. This problem occurs most often with rice, because it is often thoroughly rinsed prior to cooking, a procedure that can result in a reduction of up to 50 percent of the nutrients that were sprayed on.[85]

NUTRIENT	NUTRIENT COMPARISON	
	Whole Wheat Flour	Enriched White Flour
FIBER	11.6 g	3.5 g
CALCIUM	50 mg	20 mg
PHOSPHORUS	445 mg	100 mg
MAGNESIUM	135 mg	30 mg
ZINC	2.9 mg	0.8 mg
VITAMIN B$_6$	1.1 mg	0.07 mg
PANTOTHENIC ACID	1.3 mg	0.5 mg
FOLIC ACID	46 mcg	20 mcg

Nutrient comparison of one cup whole wheat flour and one cup enriched white flour.

The best way to eat grains is in their whole and natural form. This way you will be assured of receiving all the naturally occurring nutrients as well as the health-promoting bran. Let's look at the numerous grains you have to choose from.

AMARANTH

Amaranth's history dates back to the Aztecs. Today it is produced largely by China and Central America. This tiny, pale yellow grain can be used like wheat. In cooking, you can split a wheat-flour measurement, using half amaranth and half wheat flour. Amaranth has a high protein content and is richer in calcium than any other grain.

BARLEY

Barley was first cultivated in China around 2000 B.C.. Today, the most popular form of barley is an ivory-colored form called "pearled barley," which has had its bran removed. The most nutritious form is "hulled barley," in which the bran is left intact and the fiber, iron, and calcium content remains high. Barley is also a rich source of potassium. This versatile grain can be added to soups, broth, salads, mixed with vegetables, and even made into a hot breakfast cereal.

BUCKWHEAT

Technically, buckwheat is not a grain because it is not part of the gramineae grass family. Nevertheless, this food is loaded with vitamin E, potassium, phosphorus, and B vitamins. With the exception of "buckwheat pancakes," this grain has not enjoyed much popularity in the United States, which is quite a loss. Buckwheat has a distinct taste and a rich, nutty flavor.

CORNMEAL

A staple for the Native Americans, cornmeal is made from ground corn. Like other grains, the best way to buy it is in its whole form with the germ and bran still present. While most people have had cornbread and corn muffins, this hearty grain can make terrific pancakes, as well as polenta, a dish that is increasing in popularity in the United States.

KAMUT

Once known as "King Tut's wheat," this buttery-flavored grain is a relative of modern wheat. Kamut is higher in protein than many other grains and rich in minerals. There is an increasing number of organic kamut breads, cereals, and pastas available.

MILLET

Considered a sacred food by the Chinese, millet is high in protein, the B vitamins, copper, and iron. The grain is small and absorbs flavors well. Like barley, millet can be made into a tasty hot cereal. It can also be mixed into salads or casseroles or eaten in place of rice. Those who make their own granola at home may enjoy adding millet to the mix.

OATS

Oats contain calcium, phosphorus, iron, vitamin E, thiamin, riboflavin, and the B-vitamin complex. Although oats have been around for almost 2,000 years and have always been a primary staple in the diet of the Scottish, they didn't gain popularity in the United States until recently. This interest has been brought about by numerous publicized studies that show that oats can play an important part in lowering cholesterol levels.

Fortunately, all oats retain their bran and germ, so their fiber content is higher than grains that have been refined. Of all the grains, oats seem to be the most popular for making hot cereal (oatmeal), either *old-fashioned* or *quick-cooking*. The old-fashioned variety are whole oats that have been heated and rolled flat. Quick-cooking oats have been sliced and then heated and rolled – this process makes them cook in about a minute. Granola, which has become quite popular, is also made from oats.

Oats can be used to make healthy and hearty muffins. If you make your own breads, try adding oats to the recipe. For a heartier and flavorful pancake, add oats to your whole-wheat cakes!

QUINOA

Pronounced *keen-wah,* this staple of the Incas is quickly becoming very popular in the United States. Known as a "super-nutrient" grain, quinoa is the only grain that is a complete protein. Packed with iron, riboflavin, manganese, zinc, copper, potassium, and magnesium, it has a pale yellow color when cooked and a mild, nutty flavor. Quinoa works well mixed in most baked goods and can be a great addition to a green salad.

RICE

There are numerous varieties of rice, including long-grain, short-grain, white, brown, wehani, wild, arborio, and basmati. Although rice is the most popular grain food in the United States, we are at the bottom of the list in terms of world consumption. In Asia, the nutritional value of rice has long been known, and the grain is a primary staple of the diet.

Rice is a good source of B vitamins, iron, magnesium, and phosphorus, as well as protein. Like barley, however, the bulk of rice eaten in the United States is in the refined form of polished white rice. Conversely, brown rice retains its bran and germ and is considerably richer in vitamins, minerals, and fiber.

RYE

One of the least-well-known grains, rye is significantly higher in protein than whole wheat. It also contains B vitamins and iron. While consumed widely in Scandinavia, what little rye we eat in the United States is in the form of rye bread, which is largely refined wheat flour and rye mixed together. Rye can be added to oatmeal, breads, muffins, rice, or, in its flake form, prepared as a hot cereal or mixed in with homemade granola.

SPELT

This 5,000-year-old grain is becoming quite popular, particularly among those who have gluten and other grain allergies, because of its low gluten level. It has a nutty flavor and is rich in B vitamins. Recently, several spelt breads and bagels have been introduced by alternative baking companies.

VEGETABLES

The incidence of most types of cancer is double among people who eat few fruits and vegetables as compared to those who eat about five portions per day.
– Dr. Bruce Ames, Professor of Biochemistry and Molecular Biology
University of California, Berkeley

Vegetables contain no saturated fat or cholesterol and relatively few calories. Next to fruits, vegetables are the richest source of vitamins and minerals, particularly the important antioxidant vitamins, as well as anti-cancer phytochemicals. Would you believe that a green pepper has more vitamin C than an orange? A red pepper has almost three times as much vitamin C as an orange.

VEGETABLES AND PHYTOCHEMICALS

While it is clear that cancer rates are lower among those who eat greater amounts of fruits and vegetables, scientists are now gaining a better understanding of why. Their attention has been focused upon the non-nutrient compounds in plants known as phytochemicals (*phyto* meaning "plant").

Phytochemicals work in a variety of ways that can help protect us from various forms of cancer. Some block carcinogenic agents from forming in the first place, others prevent carcinogens from reaching target cells, and still others stimulate the production of powerful enzymes that can disarm carcinogens.[86]

While there are literally hundreds of phytochemicals, certain ones have been getting a great deal of attention for their anti-cancer properties. These include genistein (found in cabbage and soy), glucobrassicin (found in cauliflower and Brussel sprouts), indole-3-carbinols (found in broccoli), sulphoraphane (found in turnips and cabbage), and the organosulfer compounds (found in garlic, onions, and leeks).

VEGETABLES AND CAROTENOIDS

Also of significance in disease prevention are the carotenoid-rich vegetables – those red, yellow, and orange vegetables such as carrots, tomatoes, and squash. Carotenoids are pigments that exist in all plants. In green-leafed plants, the pigments are hidden by chlorophyll until autumn, when the season brings out these vibrant hues. Carotenoids play an important role in protecting plants from damage caused by oxygen and the sun's ultraviolet rays. It is now understood that carotenoids have the same protective effect in humans.

In Chapter Seven, The Micronutrients, we looked at beta carotene, the precursor to vitamin A and the most well-known carotenoid of all. There are many other important members of the carotenoid family, including alpha carotene, gamma carotene, lutein and phycotene.

Like the antioxidant vitamins C and E, carotenoids have the ability to protect human cells from free-radical and oxidative damage. We know that those who consume a carotenoid-rich diet have a greater tolerance for the sun's ultraviolet rays than those who don't. We also know that carotenoids can help prevent oxidation of lipids or fats, a process known to contribute to atherosclerosis. Studies have shown that carotenoids help to protect lymphocytes, macrophages, and natural killer cells, all important defense cells of the immune system. It has also been found that high levels of carotenoids from whole foods may retard the progression of, and may prevent, some forms of cancer.[87]

Although there is an incredible array of colorful vegetables available to us, many people rarely venture away from carrots and potatoes. Remember, the key to Whole Health is to include a *wide variety* of healthful and delicious vegetables.

LEGUMES

A legume is a plant that bears seeds enclosed in pods that split upon maturity. We eat these pods in the form of beans, peas, and lentils. Legumes are probably the oldest crop in the world. Some evidence has indicated that they may have been an important crop as far back as 10,000 years ago. Today legumes make up a substantial part of the diet of people in Asia, Latin America, the Middle East, and India.

Until recently legumes were an ignored food source in America. They have been called the "poor man's protein." The truth is that they are an outstanding, inexpensive, and very versatile food that not only provides a significant amount of protein (12-20 grams per cup) and fiber (6-8 grams per cup), but also a substantial supply of the B vitamins, calcium, magnesium, iron, potassium, and zinc, as well as several anti-cancer phytochemicals. Another wonderful quality of beans is that they are extremely durable and store well. Stored in a well-sealed container and in a dry place, beans can be kept for up to a year.

Most varieties of legumes are delicious eaten alone or as a side dish, added to soups or chilies, combined with rice, or mixed in with a variety of vegetables. One of the reasons that legumes have not been as popular as they could be is the myth that they are difficult to cook. On the contrary, legumes are one of the easiest foods to prepare. In Chapter Fourteen, you will find a guide for cooking a variety of legumes, and an excellent recipe, Middle Eastern Lentils.

SOY FOODS

Recently it has been shown that tofu and other soy foods not only contain the previously mentioned phytochemicals — including isoflavones, genistein, protease inhibitors, and phytic acids — that provide protection from heart disease and certain forms of cancer, but numerous studies have demonstrated the cholesterol-lowering effect of soy. One recent study in the *New England Journal of Medicine* demonstrated, in some cases, a reduction of up to 20 percent in a month! Such a drop in cholesterol levels almost equals a 30 percent reduction in risk of coronary heart disease. What's more, it seems that soy foods have the effect of lowering LDL ("bad") cholesterol while not adversely affecting HDL ("good") cholesterol.[88]

TOFU

Although tofu has been around for over 1,000 years in parts of Asia, we are just beginning to understand the nutritional value of this versatile food in the West. Tofu has recently been called a "miracle food" because of the many benefits researchers are just now discovering about this product and other soy foods. Ironically, the United States is the largest producer of soy beans (which are used to make tofu), yet we export the majority of it to other countries.

Tofu falls under the legume category and is made by curding soybean milk. Not only is it a good source of complete protein (it contains all of the essential amino acids), but tofu contains no cholesterol, and, when made with calcium sulfate, is an excellent source of calcium. Furthermore, it's very affordable! While regular tofu does contain a fair amount of fat, it is unsaturated. There are a few brands of *silken* tofu, such as Mori-Nu,® that contain only a few grams of fat.

Tofu works well in almost any dish, particularly those in which you might normally include meat or poultry, such as curries or pastas; it also does wonders for homemade salad dressings. An added benefit is that many brands of tofu are made from organic soybeans.

TEMPEH

Tempeh (pronounced *tem-pay*) is another food derived from fermented soybeans and occasionally grains. It is very popular in Indonesia. It has a nutty flavor and unique texture that makes it a good replacement for meat in chili and for grilling or steaming, as well as a tasty addition to vegetable sautés and pasta dishes. There are also a number of tempeh burgers on the market. Tempeh is found either refrigerated, usually along with tofu, or sometimes frozen.

TEXTURIZED VEGETABLE PROTEIN (TVP)

TVP is made from defatted soy flour that has been compressed until it takes on a flake texture. Once rehydrated, TVP works wonders in replacing the meat normally found in dishes such as chili, sloppy joes, hamburgers, and hot dogs.

SOY FLOUR

Soy flour is made from roasted soybeans that have been ground into a fine powder. Available in full-fat and defatted versions, soy flour is heavier than wheat flour. For this reason it is best to limit it to 15 – 20 percent of a recipe's flour requirement. It can also be added to gravies and sauces.

SOY MILK

Soy milk is made by pressing soaked and cooked soybeans with water. The result is a creamy milk-like beverage with a nutty flavor, that can be used in a variety of ways. Soy milk works well with cold and hot cereals, in soups and sauces, pancakes, and other recipes that call for milk. Aside from its supply of protein and B vitamins, most soy milks are fortified with vitamins A and D, calcium, and at least one company offers vitamin B_{12} fortification.

FRUIT

Aside from the wonderfully sweet tastes they offer, fruits, along with vegetables, are one of the primary sources of the cancer preventative antioxidants and phytochemicals discussed earlier. Again, those who consume five servings of fruits and vegetables a day cut their cancer risk by about 50 percent. Fruit is rich in vitamins (particularly A and C), minerals (magnesium, copper, and manganese), and high in fiber. One medium orange contains over 60 mg of vitamin C. One cup of raisins contains 102 mg of calcium.

The sweetness of fruit comes from a natural form of sugar, unlike the sugars found in many processed sweets such as cookies, candies, and soft drinks, and it provides the body with a more balanced supply of energy. Most fruits are also good sources of fiber, particularly if they are eaten with their skins on (except bananas, of course). Those fruits highest in fiber are apples, apricots, oranges, bananas, peaches, pears, and raisins. Fruits also contain a high quantity of water, something most of us could use more of in our diet.

Some individuals experience digestive difficulties when they combine fruit with other foods. If you have this experience, make a point of eating your fruits separately, such as early in the morning at least a half-hour before breakfast and as between-meal snacks.

NUTS AND SEEDS

Nuts and seeds are nutrient-dense, and a few, such as almonds and filberts, are a good source of calcium. Almonds also contain the anti-cancer phytochemicals genistein and protease inhibitors. Flaxseeds contain genistein and lignans and ferulic acid. Pumpkin seeds contain essential fatty acids and iron. Walnuts contain ellagic acid, which also has anti-cancer properties. However, all nuts and seeds are naturally high in fat. For this reason, their consumption should be limited. They can be enjoyed on occasion in a handful portion, sprinkled over a salad, or mixed in with a vegetable sauté. What you want to avoid is sitting down with a container of oil-roasted nuts and devouring them in front of the TV. Nuts and seeds don't make meals; but they can complement them.

Nuts and seeds that have been roasted not only have a higher fat content, but, for some people, are more difficult to digest. Furthermore, the oils used to roast nuts are often rancid. Roasting may also destroy the B-complex vitamins contained in nuts.

The best way to enjoy these treats is in their raw form. Because cracked nuts or nut pieces are more vulnerable to deterioration, they often have a more chewy than crunchy consistency if they are not especially fresh. For the highest nutritional quality and an extended shelf-life, it is best to buy organic nuts and seeds in their whole and raw form, in the shell when possible, and to keep them refrigerated.

Note: Peanuts are susceptible to natural molds that produce what are thought to be carcinogenic aflatoxins. Since "the jury is still out" regarding this, I suggest you look for organically grown peanuts that have been "sun dried." When the nuts are dried this way the risk of the mold developing is eliminated.

FOOD GROUP	THE REVISED AMERICAN DIET™	
	Servings per day	Serving size
WHOLE GRAINS breads/cereals	6 or more	1/2 cup oats 1/2 cup brown rice 1 cup whole-wheat pasta 1 cup cereal 1 slice bread
VEGETABLES green other yellow/red/orange	1-2 1-2 1-2	1 cup broccoli (cooked) 1 cup carrots (cooked) 1 cup spinach/collards/kale 1 medium baked potato
LEGUMES	2-3	1/2 cup lentils (cooked) 1/2 cup black beans (cooked) 1 cup tofu 1 cup fortified soy milk
FRUITS	2-4	1 medium apple 1/2 cup chopped fruit 1/2 cup berries 1/4 cup dried fruit

Number of servings and serving sizes are provided as an initial guide. You need not be overly concerned with exact portions of whole grains, vegetables, legumes, and fruits. Some highly active individuals, such as athletes, may need more servings to maintain their body weight.

FOOD GROUP	EXAMPLES FROM THE FOUR FOOD GROUPS
WHOLE GRAINS	Amaranth, barley, buckwheat, bulgur, quinoa, millet, rye, triticale, pasta, cereals (oatmeal, granola and shredded wheat), breads, tortillas, corn, popcorn, cornmeal, cornflour, brown rice, oats, spelt, kamut.
VEGETABLES	Artichokes, asparagus, bamboo shoots, beets, broccoli, Brussel sprouts, cabbage, carrots, cauliflower, chard, cucumber, garlic, eggplant, jica-ma, kale, leeks, parsley, sprouts, lettuce, peas, peppers, pumpkin, onions, tomatoes, mushrooms, potatoes, spinach, squash, yams.
LEGUMES	Adzuki beans, black beans, cranberry beans, fava beans, flageolets, Great Northern beans, kidney beans, lima beans, mung beans, navy beans, pinto beans, red beans, soybeans, black-eyed peas, chickpeas, red lentils, green split peas, yellow split peas, brown lentils, green lentils, tempeh, tofu, soy milk.
FRUITS	Apples, blackberries, cranberries, guavas, mangoes, peaches, pineap-ples, apricots, blueberries, figs, kiwis, melons, pears, raisins, bananas, boysenberries, grapefruits, lemons, oranges, plums, raspberries, dates, cherries, limes, papayas, prunes, strawberries.

GENERAL GUIDELINES FOR THE REVISED AMERICAN DIET

1. Choose fresh foods in place of boxed, canned, and packaged foods as often as possible.

No matter how you look at it, foods that have been packaged, boxed, or canned are nutritionally inferior to fresh foods. The ways in which packaged foods are processed and then stored significantly depletes the vitamins and minerals they originally contained. Foods that are packaged also often contain high levels of fats and numerous additives such as coloring, texturizers, flavor enhancers, emulsifiers, and excess sodium, as well as preservatives to maintain their shelf life. The human body has no use for these additives and has difficulty eliminating many of them. In addition, some individuals may have allergic reactions to these additives. Make fresh, whole foods your first choice. When packaged foods are necessary, be sure to choose those without preservatives and other additives.

2. Avoid refined sugar.

Those who follow the Standard American Diet are getting about 33 teaspoons of sugar a day! That amounts to about 525 calories of a product that damages our health.

You now know that refined carbohydrates are poor sources of energy. Sugar is a form of carbohydrate, but in an extremely refined form. Thus, when it is ingested, it may be incorporated into the bloodstream rapidly. Normally, in a balanced state, our bloodstream contains about a teaspoon of sugar. Amounts above this begin to create an imbalance. Along with placing a strain on the pancreas, energy is required to eliminate the excess sugar. Sugar has been implicated in the onset of tooth decay, suppression of immune function, diabetes, and obesity.

Probably the most convincing reason to cut back, if not eliminate, sugar from the diet entirely is the fact that sugar has been shown to interfere with the functioning of the immune system.[89] In one study, the ability of white blood cells to attack invading bacteria was suppressed for up to five hours after consumption of five teaspoons of sugar.[90] Now consider that the average cola soft drink contains 12 teaspoons of sugar! It would be a challenge to get someone to ingest 12 teaspoons of sugar, spoon by spoon. On the other hand, most people would have no problem with drinking two cola drinks (24 teaspoons of sugar).

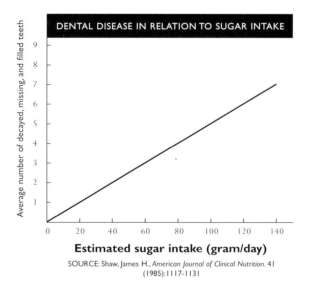

SOURCE: Shaw, James H., *American Journal of Clinical Nutrition.* 41
(1985):1117-1131

SUGAR AND YOUR TEETH

Tooth decay is a pervasive problem in the United States and it is due primarily to the quantity of sugar consumed. The latest U.S. Department of Agriculture survey found that nine of every ten persons suffers from some dental problem, including missing teeth, decayed teeth (cavities), and periodontal disease. Sugar feeds the bacteria in the mouth that cause tooth decay. The bacteria actually create a corrosive acid that eats away at tooth enamel, so as we increase our intake of sugar, we make the acid's job of destruction easier. For anyone who doubts the link between tooth decay and sugar consumption, consider that during World Wars I and II, when there were drastic shortages of sugar, tooth decay rates dropped markedly.

SUGAR IS COMPOSED OF EMPTY CALORIES.

The term "empty calories" refers to the lack of nutrients in sugar. Although a form of carbohydrate, sugar offers nothing of nutritional value to your diet. Sugar, and the nutrient-deficient foods it is often included in, takes the place of more healthful and nutrient-dense foods. High-sugar foods often promote nutrient deficiencies when they make up a large part of the diet.

3. Use sodium in moderation or not at all.

Most of the sodium we consume is artificially added to our diet. Less than 10 percent of our sodium intake occurs naturally in the foods we eat.[91] A significant amount of the sodium we consume comes from the salt shaker in the form of sodium chloride (table salt is 40 percent sodium and 60 percent chloride). The remainder is contained in processed foods. For flavor, texture, and preservation, varying amounts of salt are added to many processed foods, from salad dressings to pickles to chicken broth. Smoked meats (hams, bacon, sausage) and fish, as well as canned foods (particularly soups) and snack foods, such as pretzels and potato chips, are all very high in sodium. Several sodium compounds are also often found in processed foods, including sodium benzoate (a preservative), disodium phosphate (reduces cooking time), sodium citrate (enhances flavor), and monosodium glutamate (MSG, a seasoning). Even many common over-the-counter medicines, as well as some prescription drugs, have significant levels of sodium. For this reason, it's easy for our sodium intake to soar past the recommended daily intake. An ounce of pretzels contains 500 mg of sodium. Three ounces of ham has about 1,000 mg of sodium. A fast-food cheeseburger rings up another 1,200 mg. An average dill pickle packs a whopping 1,900 mg!

In addition to raising blood pressure, excess sodium has been implicated in the development of stomach cancer. When worldwide rates for stomach cancer are graphed, it becomes clear that those populations with the highest intake of sodium also have the highest rates of stomach cancer. Although in many other respects the eating habits of the Japanese are healthy, their salt intake is enormous and ranks them as number one for stomach cancer. Their high intake is due mostly to the amount of soy sauce and pickled vegetables they eat.

HOW MUCH SODIUM DO WE NEED?

Although the human body can function perfectly on 500 mg of sodium a day, providing for varying levels of activity and climatic differences, the RDA has been set at 1,100-3,300 mg a day. In reality, the average diet contains somewhere between 3,000 and 6,000 mg a day, about 2,000 mg of which is added at the dining table.[92] By far, the most effective way to keep your sodium intake within the safe range is to remove the saltshaker from your table. Many people sprinkle a little table salt on everything simply out of habit. Yet just one teaspoon of table salt yields 2,000 mg of sodium! Read labels for sodium content, and watch food labels for monosodium glutamate, sodium phosphate, sodium nitrate, sodium ascorbate, baking soda, baking powder, and sodium saccharin, since all these additives contain high levels of sodium.

A taste for salt is a learned one, and so it can be unlearned as well. In place of salt as a seasoning, try some of the following spices: basil, garlic, garlic powder (not garlic salt), dill weed, ginger, rosemary, bay leaves, cloves, cumin, sage, tarragon, and curry powder.

4. Choose organic foods whenever possible.

Organic foods are those which have been grown without the use of harmful synthetic chemical pesticides, herbicides, and fertilizers. For a food to be certified organic, it must have been grown on farmland that has been free of such chemicals for a minimum of three years.

Whenever possible, choose organic fruits and vegetables. Organic farming, the most preferable alternative in terms of consumer and environmental safety, is becoming a popular and viable method for smaller farms.

When foods are grown conventionally, they are subjected to enormous quantities of harmful chemicals, many of which have not been tested for safety, some of which are known carcinogens. In my home state of California, farmers annually use nearly 400 million pounds of pesticides, about two-thirds of the annual use in this country.[93] According to a report by the National Academy of Sciences, chemical pesticides may cause an additional 1.4 million cases of cancer in America. Some of the more deadly pesticides that have been banned from use in the United States are now exported to South and Central America. Between 1992-1994, over 45 million pounds of restricted pesticides known to have "very high toxicities and environmental hazards" were exported for use outside of the United States,[94] and some of the recipients of this toxic cargo are increasingly supplying the United States with produce. By permitting this it would seem that the government is saying, "It's okay to poison Americans with known carcinogenic chemicals as long as the chemicals are applied in another country."

While some supermarket chains have attempted to assure their customers by claiming not to sell produce with detectable residues, random samplings show that the risk is still pervasive. For example, Richard Wiles of the Washington-based Environmental Working Group examined data for a three-year period and found that over 80 percent of peach, apple, and celery samples contained residues of one or more pesticides. As many as eight different pesticides were detected on a single apple.[95] In these residues, 12 known carcinogens, 17 neurotoxins, and 11 pesticides that interfere with the endocrine and reproductive systems were identified.

A more recent Food and Drug Administration study found pesticide residues in 48 percent of fruits and vegetables tested.[96] Currently, the FDA checks only 1 percent of all imported produce for pesticide residues.

Chemical pesticides reach us in more ways than one. Although much of the chemical run-off permeates our farming soils, where it remains for years, pesticides have made their way into our groundwater, lakes, and streams. Also, much of the livestock raised for human consumption feeds from pesticide-tainted grains. The animal's body accumulates these chemicals in its fat, and eventually the animal is processed for human consumption.

Not only are organic foods free from potentially carcinogenic toxins, but they also have a higher nutritional value. At Rutgers University, researchers studied the mineral quality of conventional produce (produce subjected to modern farming methods) and organic produce (produce grown in rich soils, using proper crop rotation and without the use of harmful agrichemicals). The organic produce was found, on average, to have an 87 percent higher content of magnesium, potassium, manganese, iron, and copper.[97]

Organic farming is more labor-intensive than conventional farming, which uses extensive chemicals. For this reason, organic foods tend to cost more and are not yet as available as conventionally grown foods. However, I am sure you agree that the slightly higher price is well worth the assurance that you are getting a certified chemical-, pesticide-, and irradiation-free food! Furthermore, you will undoubtedly find that your overall grocery bill will shrink considerably once you eliminate costly animal products from your shopping list.

As the demand for organic produce has increased, some of the conventional supermarkets have begun to stock various organic fruits and vegetables. Better yet, there are an increasing number of new markets opening up (see Appendix) that

5.   Read food labels.

Reading food labels is another step in taking responsibility for your health. By law, ingredient labels are supposed to list all substances included in a packaged food. Ingredients will be listed in descending order according to concentration. In other words, the ingredient that appears first in the list makes up the largest portion of the food. So if sugar is the first ingredient, you know the product is going to be extremely sweet. Sometimes a product may contain significant amounts of sweeteners that are not labeled as "sugars." For instance, Sucanat fructose, maltose, sucrose, corn syrup, high-fructose corn syrup, honey, maple syrup, and molasses are all forms of sugar.

When reading an ingredient label, be on the lookout for additives. Additives are things a food packager may include in the product to enhance its appearance and taste or extend its shelf life, but which we know our body would prefer to do without. For instance, consider a jar of peanut butter. If you pick up a jar of a famous national brand and read its ingredient label, you will find there is a lot more in the jar than peanuts, including a considerable amount of sugar. Why would anyone sweeten peanut butter? The reality is that it is done. Once you start reading labels carefully, you will see that food producers pack a lot of sugar and salt into foods you wouldn't expect. Unfortunately, sugar and salt are not your worst concerns when it comes to additives. Ingredients such as monosodium glutamate (MSG), benzoates, FD&C Yellow No. 5 (also known as tartrazine), butylated hydroxytoluene (BHT), and butylated hydrozyanisole (BHA) have all been implicated in allergic reactions that include swelling, rash, asthma, headaches, hives, and a runny nose.[98] So take a moment and compare what is available. When you look, you will find that there are several respectable brands of peanut butter that are made of nothing other than raw, crushed peanuts. Better yet, in most natural foods markets you can freshly grind nut butters.

Take a look at the ingredient label of your favorite bread. You might be surprised to find hydrogenated oil listed as an ingredient. Again, there are plenty of nutritious, whole-grain breads without this dangerous and unnecessary additive. When you come across ingredients you can't even pronounce, it's probably a good idea to put the food back on the shelf.

COMMON FOOD ADDITIVES TO AVOID

Artificial Color

It is not uncommon for artificial colors to cause allergic reactions in some people. It is believed that the coloring Yellow No. 5 can temporarily worsen the condition of asthmatics. According to the Center for Science in the Public Interest (CSPI), Blue No. 1 and No. 2, Green No. 3, and Red No. 3 have all been linked to cancer in laboratory animals.

Aspartame

A sweetener manufactured from methanol (wood alcohol) and two amino acids, Aspartame is sold under the names Equal® and Nutrasweet®, and has been linked to literally thousands of problems. In fact, the FDA has logged over 3,000 complaints about this product, with symptoms including headache, numbness, dizziness, nausea, depression, and vision problems. Those who suffer from phenylketonuria (PKU), individuals who cannot break down the amino acid phenylalanine, must avoid this product.

Butylated Hydroxyanisole (BHA)

BHA is a preservative that is commonly found in packaged foods, including baked goods, soups, potato flakes, breakfast cereals, and chewing gum. This product may have adverse affects on the nervous system.

Butylated Hydroxytoluene (BHT)

BHT is used similarly to BHA. It is believed to be toxic to the kidneys, and has the additional risk of being a suspected carcinogen. England has already banned the use of this additive.

Caseinate

This is a milk protein used to enhance texture. Therefore, when avoiding dairy products be sure to look for this ingredient. It is typically used in frozen desserts, but you may also find it in non-dairy creamers and a few soy cheeses.

Monosodium Glutamate (MSG)

MSG is a flavor enhancer that occurs in both a natural and synthetic form. It has been linked to a host of reactions in those who are sensitive to it, including migraine headache, rash, nausea, ringing in the ears, elevated blood pressure, bronchospasms, and dizziness. Those who have asthma are at increased risk. Because in the past MSG was commonly used in Chinese restaurants, the reactions were termed "Chinese Restaurant Syndrome." MSG is sold under the trade name Accent in supermarkets.

Mono- and Diglycerides

These are chemical preservatives commonly used in breads, frozen desserts, margarine, conventional peanut butters, and numerous baked goods. They are currently being studied for adverse reproductive effects.

Propyl Gallate

A preservative used similarly to BHA and BHT, this additive may cause stomach and skin irritation and is a suspected carcinogen. It is used in ice cream, some fruit drinks, candy, and gelatin desserts. Those who have asthma are particularly sensitive to it.

Saccharin

Saccharin is an artificial sweetener that the FDA has considered banning for some time. A known carcinogen, it still shows up in some soft drinks and in Sweet 'N Low® brand sweetener.

Sodium Nitrite

Commonly used in bacon, ham, smoked fish, and sandwich meats, this preservative is a known carcinogen.

CHAPTER ELEVEN

SPECIAL CONCERNS

*Forty percent of American children ages 5-8 are obese, or
have elevated cholesterol or high blood pressure.*
– President's Council on Physical Fitness and Sports

CHILDREN AND THE REVISED AMERICAN DIET

Some adults who have made the transition to the Revised American Diet still have reservations when considering their children's diet. Many of parents' fears have little basis in reality, however. The truth is, once an infant is weaned from breast milk and begins eating a variety of solid foods, there is no reason whatsoever that they should consume any of the foods with excessive saturated fat, cholesterol, protein, and sodium found in the average child's diet. The Revised American Diet, composed of grains, legumes, fruits, vegetables, nuts, and seeds, will provide all the necessary nutrients a child needs to develop in a healthy and sound manner – perhaps, as we will see, a manner superior to that of their meat-eating counterparts.

We live in a time when the average child's blood cholesterol level is dangerously high. As we now know, the ravages of heart disease begin early in life. Children younger than 10 years have been found to have arterial plaque already developing. Further, each year about 1,000 teenagers will suffer a stroke caused by the symptoms of a high-fat diet, high blood pressure, and atherosclerosis. When we look at the types and quantities of foods being consumed by the average child today, such cases of disease are not so surprising. It is not just the foods that children eat at home. The average school menu is a nutritional disaster. A recent report by the USDA brings home the alarming lack of nutrition provided to children by schools today. The

60 percent whey and 40 percent curd. Cow's milk, however, contains about 80 percent curd. This is fine for a baby calf, but human infants have difficulty digesting so much curd. Breast milk has a greater percentage of unsaturated fat as well.

A protein in cow's milk, IgG, has been implicated in colic, a condition in which infants spit up continually and produce a high-pitched scream. Even in infants where dairy is avoided, colic remains a risk if the mother ingests dairy products. This is because the protein will end up in her breast milk (contaminating her milk for up to 10 days after ingestion), and ultimately be passed on to the nursing infant, eliciting an allergic reaction.[99]

Dairy products are one of the leading sources of delayed food allergies and may cause a variety of symptoms including skin rash, diarrhea, gas, bloating, runny nose, and headache.

Another major concern is the condition mentioned earlier known as lactose intolerance. At about four years of age, the body *naturally* stops producing the digestive enzyme lactase. In the absence of lactase, the sugar in milk, lactose, cannot be digested. When a child or adult without this enzyme consumes milk and other dairy products, he will often experience gas, abdominal cramping, and diarrhea. This often overlooked condition is widespread, and a child can be spared the misery it brings simply by not introducing dairy products to their diet. Again, I want to stress that lactose intolerance is a natural process. As nature intended, when a child is weaned from the breast, there is no need for the body to produce this lactase any longer. Children who are able to continue digesting milk sugar are the exception rather than the norm.

Infants younger than two who are fed cow's milk often experience gastrointestinal bleeding, which ultimately can lead to iron-deficiency anemia.[100] Frank Oski, M.D., director of the Department of Pediatrics at Johns Hopkins University School of Medicine, and physician in chief at Johns Hopkins Children's Center, explains that this sensitivity to cow's milk "rarely produces dramatic symptoms but results in slow and steady bleeding. Infants with this form of milk sensitivity may lose 1 to 5 milliliters of blood per day in their stool…from this steady hemorrhage. The volumes of blood lost each day are too small for detection by simple visual examination…the blood can only be detected by chemical tests." The latest estimates are that 15 to 20 percent of children under two years of age suffer from iron-deficiency anemia and that at least half of the cases can be attributed to this gastrointestinal bleeding. Research has demonstrated that this iron loss can be significant enough to interfere with brain development and, ultimately, future intelligence.[101] A study reported in the February 1992 issue of the medical journal *The Lancet* supports this theory. In the study, which involved 300 children, it was found that infants who were fed mother's milk "had a significantly higher I.Q." At eight years of age, those children who received only mother's milk had I.Q.s 10 percent higher than those children fed cow's milk.

Not only do vegetarian children demonstrate equal or higher intelligence in some cases, they grow up to be just as tall and as strong as children raised on the Standard American Diet. The only real difference between vegetarian children and non-vegetarian children is that vegetarians are not overweight. A lean child is something every parent can feel good about, particularly since the American Heart Association states that obesity in children ages six to eleven has increased 54 percent since 1963.

If this is not enough evidence why children should not be given dairy products, it has also been found that infants who are given cow's milk run twice the risk of dying from Sudden Infant Death Syndrome (SIDS).[102] An important study in *Clinical and Experimental Allergy* has implicated an allergic reaction to cow's milk as one of the causes of SIDS. The study indicates that when infants who are allergic to cow's milk are given the substance prior to sleeping, they may experience an allergic reaction during sleep. The reaction, anaphylaxis, may result in the infant regurgitating and then inhaling that regurgitation into the lungs, which then causes shock and sudden death.

Again, the very best food for an infant is breast milk from its mother. Breast milk is loaded with all of the vitamins, minerals, and other nutrients necessary for proper growth. Ideally, breast feeding should continue for the first year of life. If for some reason the mother is unable to provide the infant with breast milk, she should substitute a fortified soy-based formula. There are several brands available that are prepared without the use of animal products.

VITAMIN B$_{12}$

As we discussed earlier, vitamin B$_{12}$ is required by the body. In planning their child's diet, parents should be sure their child is receiving an adequate supply. At about six months, the infant can be given a liquid B$_{12}$ supplement. After the infant has started consuming solid foods, several fortified foods can be relied upon for the vitamin. Soon, soy milks will be fortified with B$_{12}$, but, to be certain, read the label. Breakfast cereals are also often fortified with B$_{12}$; again read the labels to be sure. Finally, after the first year, fortified nutritional yeast can also be used to assure a good supply. Prior to the first year, nucleic acids in the yeast may be challenging for the infant's kidneys. Nutritional yeast can be added to most foods, including salads, soups, vegetable sautés, and more, and is quite flavorful.

OTHER VITAMIN SUPPLEMENTS

Aside from all the evidence that indicates a child provided with a well-balanced vegan diet does not need any vitamin supplementation (with the possible exception of vitamin B$_{12}$), some parents still feel better employing this form of insurance. As long as the vitamin supplement does not exceed the U.S. Recommended Daily Allowance, it should not pose a problem. There are several brands of vegetarian multivitamins specifically prepared for children that can be found at a well-stocked natural foods market or health food store. Since children often resist swallowing vitamin tablets, the best approach is to crush them into a powder and add them to soup, apple sauce, or mashed potatoes, or use a liquid multivitamin preparation.

When considering the advantages of a vegetarian diet for children, rate of development is one area that has been largely overlooked. Children today are maturing at a much faster rate than ever before, and experts are pointing at the level of fat consumption. The reason is that high fat levels promote high levels of both sex and growth hormones. This is of particular concern for girls. While prior to the turn of the century, the average age of menarche (first menstruation) was 17, it is now 12.5 years of age. Even in Japan, where fat consumption has been traditionally low but has been steadily climbing with the Western influence on diet, the average age at which girls enter puberty has dropped from 15.2 to 12.5 years of age in only the last four decades.[103] Yet according to Cornell University biochemist and director of the China Health Study Dr. T. Colin Campbell, in China, where fat consumption is still among the lowest in the world, girls reach puberty between 15 and 19 years of age.

Studies show that women who reached menarche before age 13 have a 4.2 times higher risk of developing breast cancer later in life. In addition to this increased risk, it simply seems unfair that mere children are having to contend with the many issues and responsibilities associated with a woman's body.

Vegetarian children will mature more slowly, the way nature intended them to, their adult teeth will come in later, and females will begin menstruating later, providing them with added protection against the current high incidence of breast cancer. Vegetarian children will grow to be just as tall, strong, and attractive as their peers, if not more so, yet they will be free of the various allergies and chronic diseases that afflict so many of their non-vegetarian counterparts.

FEEDING GUIDE

Infants (0-1 year)

Breast feeding for at least the first year.

Soy-based formula when breast feeding is not possible.*

At 4-6 months, solid foods can be introduced, one at a time.

Include vegetables, fruits, fortified cereals, tofu, and soy yogurt.

Liquid B_{12} supplement may be used at 6 months.

At 7-8 months, beans, peas, and lentils (well mashed) may be introduced.

Toddlers (2-4 years)

Fortified full-fat soy milk beverage remains important in the diet.

Breads and other grains may be included.

Nut butters such as cashew, almond, and tahini may be used.

Children (5-11 years)

Food types remain the same, yet serving size begins to equal adult's.

Children's food intake will vary according to activity level and should not
  be restricted unless excessive weight becomes evident.

Variety in food choices is key.

* Soy milk products not prepared especially for infants do not contain necessary methionine, vitamins, and iron. Be sure it is an infant formula.

PREGNANCY AND THE REVISED AMERICAN DIET

The diet of a pregnant mother has always been highly controversial. Conventional wisdom built upon nutritional myths has led mothers and many well-meaning physicians to believe that pregnancy requires lots of meat and dairy products to support the development of the child. Fortunately, this is only a myth. There is no more reason for a pregnant woman to consume animal products than for a woman who is not pregnant. With the exception of vitamin B_{12}, a mother-to-be can derive all the necessary nutrients to support both herself and her baby by eating plenty of whole grains, legumes, vegetables, fruits, nuts, and seeds. Pregnant women have been doing this for thousands of years, giving birth to happy and healthy infants.

PREGNANCY AND CALORIES

Pregnancy does bring an increased appetite (usually around the second trimester), as the mother is eating for both herself and her developing child. Usually, this entails an increase of about 300 calories a day. Pregnancy also increases the need for the essential fats (linoleic and linolenic acid) and iron. The essential fats are abundant in pumpkin seeds, broccoli, spinach, soy, and legumes, and flaxseed oil, as well as many nuts and their butters, which are also highly caloric. Increasing the intake of these foods will suffice.

In addition to all the unhealthy side effects of consuming high-fat animal foods, pregnant mothers on the Standard American Diet tend to gain large amounts of weight because animal products are so high in fat. The excess weight they gain not only makes pregnancy and delivery more difficult, but may also be a risk factor for both diabetes and high blood pressure. After pregnancy, the mother must contend with losing the excess weight she has gained. Vegetarian mothers, however, are much less likely to gain such significant amounts of weight during their pregnancies.

PREGNANCY AND OTHER MICRONUTRIENTS

Iron requirements for women vary because of differing rates of absorption. Some women absorb significantly more iron from the foods they eat than others. Normally, the suggested intake for iron is 18 mg a day, but pregnancy increases the requirement to the range of 30-60 mg a day, depending on how well the mother absorbs iron.

It has been found that vitamin C enhances the absorption rate of iron when the two are consumed together. For this reason, vitamin C-rich foods such as tomatoes, broccoli, and bell peppers may be combined with iron-rich food sources. Iron-rich foods include dried fruits, such as raisins and apricots, leafy greens, whole grains, legumes, nuts, and seeds. However, because iron deficiency is not uncommon among women, the best advice for a pregnant mother is to consult her physician and have a ferritin blood test to determine her iron level.

It should be encouraging to know that a 1990 report by the Institute of Medicine, National Academy of Sciences, indicated that vegetarian mothers-to-be

enter a market. Throughout the day, we are exposed to numerous restaurants, catering trucks with a parade of food, delivery services that bring meals to our home or office, and vending machines that offer everything from soup to sandwiches.

With this abundance and immediate availability of food, it becomes rather easy to lose sight of how it reaches us, and at what cost (aside from the financial one). Yet when we are faced with scarcity, we become far more sensitive to where our supplies are coming from and how they reach us. The fact that you are reading this book would suggest that you probably don't know what it's like to have to climb a tree to pick your fruit, or venture across a hot desert or into a thick forest for days to trap your family's next meal. Hopefully, it also means that you've never had to sit on a street corner or in a back alley and beg passersby for your next meal.

One man who has given a great deal of thought to what is involved in the production of the foods (specifically the meat-centered diet) that feed the developed nations of the world is John Robbins. He is the author of *Diet for a New America* and *May All Be Fed: Diet for a New World*, as well as the founder of the EarthSave Foundation in Santa Cruz, California. Not only did Mr. Robbins give a great deal of thought to the processes of food production, but he also researched and documented his findings in the two compelling and sobering books mentioned above. In his works, Mr. Robbins demonstrates that it is, in fact, the meat-centered diet that is largely responsible not only for the consumption of enormous amounts of our natural resources, but for the polluting and toxification of them as well. Most of us are ignorant of what is required to produce the quantities of beef, chicken, eggs, and milk that are consumed daily in this country, and understandably so. When was the last time any of us visited a dairy farm, cattle ranch, or slaughterhouse? To learn more, I encourage you to read both of Mr. Robbins's excellent books. They are extremely informative and beautifully written in a manner that will likely change the way you think about food and our natural resources forever. I would like to present some facts to you that are derived from the research presented in *Diet for a New America* and another EarthSave publication, *Realities for the '90s*. I know that these facts will be further inspiration for you to make the wisest decisions about the foods you and your family choose to eat.

The process through which beef, chicken, and dairy products are produced is the most costly, inefficient, and wasteful—not to mention cruel—one in the world. It is a process that consumes enormous resources, including water, fossil fuels, vital trees, insects, plants, and animals, at a rate that the earth simply can no longer accommodate. It is a process that not only exposes us all to numerous hazardous chemicals, drugs, and pollutants, but one that makes misery of the lives of millions of animals everyday. The costs of this consumption are showing up in everyday life and with increasing urgency.

Each day in America 130,000 cattle, 7,000 calves, 360,000 hogs and 24 million chickens are needlessly slaughtered. I say needlessly because it has been clearly established that humans thrive on a plant-based diet, and there is no biological need for eating animals.

In an effort to keep business profitable and efficient, all of these animals are subjected to horrifying treatments that include having their beaks chopped off (chickens), tails cut off (hogs), and confinement to stalls so small they cannot turn around or simply scratch themselves. They are injected and implanted with antibiotics, hormones and other drugs, and fed everything from cement dust to sheep brains to their own blood.

During their short lives these animals and the manner in which they are raised will take a drastic toll on the environment.

Consider the water used in the production of livestock. Earlier we looked at how essential pure water is to human health. We also learned how obtaining pure water for human consumption has become increasingly difficult due to the level of toxins deposited in our water. Not only is our water supply becoming increasingly polluted, it is shrinking rapidly. One of the primary ways in which our water supply is diminishing is in the production of livestock. In the United States at least 50 percent of the available water is devoted to the raising of livestock.

As the demand for meat increases and the number of livestock is raised to meet this demand, this percentage will only rise. Water goes not only to each 1,000 pound steer to drink, but also to irrigate the huge quantities of grain that must be grown to feed them. It is estimated that one pound of edible beef produced in California requires approximately 2,500 gallons of water. This can be contrasted to the 24 gallons of water required to raise a pound of potatoes. Also, as the number of livestock increases, as well as the volume of grain they consume, there is an inescapable by-product: mounting quantities of animal waste. So great is this waste (some 20 billion pounds a day in the United States), that the overflow can no longer be absorbed by the land and is entering our waterways, inadvertently or intentionally. The consequences are high levels of nitrates, phosphates, ammonia, and bacteria that deplete oxygen and choke our water supply.

The consequences of cattle production extend beyond our waterways, however. Livestock occupy a significant portion of our available land. In fact, half the Earth's land mass is occupied by livestock. Today, some 3 million cattle are grazing on U.S. pasture lands, consuming 1,000 pounds of precious vegetation every month. While production in the United States is significant in itself and has accounted for the clearing of nearly 250 million acres of forest, Central and South America are now producing large quantities of beef for the United States as well. Since 1987, these two areas alone have exported 300 million pounds of meat (a large majority of which went to fast-food hamburgers). The availability of land for cattle grazing and grain-feed production is more restricted in these areas. Consequently, to keep up with the demand, cattle farmers in Central America have encroached into what was formerly pristine rain forest.

A rain forest is a wonderful sanctuary for many known and undiscovered plants (many with medicinal uses), birds, insects, and animals. Yet it is a hindrance to the cattle farmer. Consequently, rain forest acreage is being burned and cleared for cattle grazing and feed production at an alarming rate. This process is known as deforestation. To date, 25 percent of the Central American rain forests have been cleared for cattle grazing. And with the loss of these important lush microsystems, many species of plant and animal life have also disappeared. The burning of forests to make way for cattle grazing also releases huge quantities of carbon dioxide into the atmosphere, some 1.4 billion tons since 1970. The rain forests are essential to the Earth's oxygen supply, and, as they are burned off, the carbon dioxide produced not only pollutes the air, reduces oxygen, and makes breathing more difficult, it also increases the atmospheric temperature, thereby contributing to global warming.

What compounds the misfortune of this process is that little of the land cleared is of any value just a few years later. Because the soil of a rain forest is meant to be protected by a canopy of lush green growth, once the plants and trees are cleared it is extremely vulnerable. Without the plant life to retain most of its mineral stores, and with the constant exposure to wind, rain, and sun, the soil is quickly eroded and unable to support any further plant life. With their now infertile grazing land, the cattle farmers move deeper into the forest, clearing new land and repeating a perpetual cycle that apparently will end only when every acre has been deforested and desertified, unless, of course, the demand for beef is reduced.

Paul Hawken, author of *The Ecology of Commerce*, succinctly summed up this cycle of destruction when he said, "When cattle ranchers clear rain forests to raise beef to sell to fast-food chains that make hamburgers to sell to Americans who have the highest rate of heart disease in the world...we can say easily that business is no longer developing the world. We have become its predator."

It is important to understand that the environmental impact of our dietary choices is not only a consequence of the enormous consumption of beef, pork, poultry, and dairy products, but extends to seafood as well. In their quest for what has been erroneously accepted as a healthy alternative to meat, Americans have joined much of the rest of the world, consuming seafood at a rate unparalleled in history. Since 1988, sales in the U.S. alone have escalated by a billion dollars. Consequently, our oceans are being "clear cut" in much the same way that the world's forests have been over the past few decades.

Using everything from ocean floor vacuum systems to sonar tracking devices to surveillance planes to netting systems large enough to envelope twelve 747 jumbo jets, the world's 37,000 fishing vessels and 13 million fishers manage to land some

90 million metric tons of sea creatures a year. This enormous harvest of sea life has sent fish populations and the aquatic environment into a high speed downward spiral.

Today, what were once two of the world's most richly populated fishing areas, the Grand Banks off of Canada and New England's Georges Banks, are now barren waters which have been closed to fishing. In coral reefs where divers use cyanide to stun large, exotic fish, elaborate living reef ecosystems become colorless aquatic graveyards, unable to support any marine life, just weeks after the poison is released.

Over 1,000 species of fish have been listed as endangered, and over 27 species have been driven to extinction already this century. In addition to the fish that are intended for harvest each year, an enormous number of non-target fish, sea birds, turtles, and dolphins, which become entangled in fishing nets, are returned to the sea, stunned or dead.

What does choosing a vegetarian lifestyle mean to the Earth and her resources? It means lessening the destruction of the global rain forests and oceans and allowing important species of plants and animals to survive. It means helping counter the current effect of global warming. It means freeing up land that is used exclusively to produce grain for livestock and making it available to inexpensively produce sustainable food products that can significantly reduce world hunger. Currently, the amount of grain produced worldwide that is given to livestock rather than people is nearly 50 percent. According to the World Health Organization, 1.3 billion people are starving on any given day. If Americans alone reduced their consumption of meat by only 10 percent, it is estimated that the land, water, and energy (including gasoline, oil, and other fuels) normally consumed to produce livestock could provide for 100 million people to be fed.

You now have a better idea of what is involved in producing the animal foods that have for so long been the center of the American diet. Here are a few more facts derived from EarthSave's *Realities for the '90s*, Michael Parenti's *Dirty Truths* and Jeremy Rifkins's *Beyond Beef* that you may wish to keep in mind:

- The 15 billion head of livestock worldwide outnumber people three to one and occupy half the world's land mass.

- Seventy percent of grain produced in the United States is fed to livestock.

- The demand for beef is the primary cause of desertification.

- Every second, 200 Americans purchase one or more hamburgers at a fast food outlet.

- No other activity has destroyed as much rain forest in Central America as cattle grazing.

- Livestock production in the United States contributes more pollution to our water than any other industry producing toxic waste.

- Eighty-five percent of the topsoil in the United States is lost from cropland, pasture, rangeland, and forestland due to raising livestock.

- One pound of beef produced in California requires approximately 2,500 gallons of water. To produce one pound of wheat requires 25 gallons of water.

- One acre of land can produce 10,000 pounds of green beans, or 30,000 pounds of carrots or 50,000 pounds of tomatoes, but yields only 250 pounds of beef.

- Every steak has the same global warming effect as a 25-mile drive in an average American car.

- Globally about 600 million tons of grain are fed to livestock, much of it to cattle.

- The nine warmest years ever recorded in the last century were during the last fifteen years.

- In the past 20 years, the world's forests have been reduced by 296 million acres.

the plant kingdom and enjoy excellent health benefits. So the closer one moves toward a totally vegetarian or vegan diet, the greater will be one's health benefits. Why compromise – make your goal excellence in health!

It is understandable that, for some people, changing lifelong eating patterns that have largely included animal products may seem an enormous challenge at first. However, as you begin to feel better, look better, have more energy, and improve your health, your new diet becomes easier and easier and, gradually, effortless.

Some people feel that the best way to make the transition to a vegetarian diet is to make a sweeping change all at once. They believe they should stop consuming all animal products on a particular day, and let that be that. For someone who has been thinking a great deal about her diet for some time and has a very strong sense of self-discipline, this may be an effective approach. If you feel ready and have the strength, I say do it. You will notice dramatic changes most rapidly. However, I also recognize that such an approach can sometimes be very challenging and less successful than a gradual adaptation. In many cases it seems more effective to make the transition a gradual one.

Sudden changes are not only challenging psychologically, but they are often a shock to the body. As an example, people who have been consuming only a minimum of fiber in their diet (about 10 grams), may experience temporary digestive problems if they suddenly consume the recommended amount of 30 grams a day. Yet, if they gradually introduce more fiber into their diet, the transition is almost always smooth.

Again, depending on your current diet, if you were to attempt to suddenly adopt everything I have presented thus far, you would likely not only feel overwhelmed, but might even panic. So don't place that kind of pressure on yourself to begin with. Many of us have been eating the same foods in the same manner for most of our lives. We have acquired the tastes we have over time and through repetition; it is through the same repetition that we can learn new eating habits that will assure us a healthy and long life. As you make these changes, be aware of the good you are doing for yourself and how you are positively affecting your health and overall feeling of well-being. As you feel better and look better, greater change will come more easily and more naturally. You may even find yourself disliking the look, smell, and appearance of animal foods after some time, much like a smoker who quits smoking suddenly becomes sensitized to and displeased by secondhand smoke in his environment.

The easiest way to make this transition is to do so gradually, adopting new habits one by one. By progressively weaning your body of those unhealthy foods it has come to expect and replacing those foods with healthier choices, you will permit adaptation and a chance to acquire new tastes, while simultaneously restoring nutritional balance. Remember, though, your goal is to ultimately eliminate unhealthy foods from your diet entirely. Here is a summary of some steps you can take in making your transition:

1. Eliminate or reduce meat, poultry, and fish.

If you don't feel ready to eliminate meat entirely, start by cutting back on both the portion size and frequency with which you eat it. First limit eating meat to no more than three times a week. When you do have meat, make it a garnish rather than the centerpiece of your meal. For example, rather than having a steak or a couple of chicken breasts, mince a bit of turkey and mix it with a larger portion of rice and vegetables. Begin incorporating tofu, tofu burgers and hot dogs, and tempeh products into your meals.

2. Eliminate or reduce dairy products.

If you are not ready to eliminate dairy entirely, begin by switching to non-fat or skim-milk products. This will cut back considerably on fat content. Remember, whole milk contains nearly 50 percent of its calories as fat. Low-fat milk has about 38 percent of its calories as fat. Many people erroneously believe that 2 percent milk is 2 percent fat. Unfortunately, this is not the case. Two-percent milk still gets

22 percent of its calories from fat. However, skim or non-fat milk contains only 4 percent of its calories from fat.

During this transition period, choose organic dairy products. Begin using soy milk, rice milk, or almond milk. These great-tasting replacements can be used just like milk on cold and hot cereals and in your favorite recipes that call for milk. Soy milks and other non-dairy beverages are sold in 8-ounce aseptic containers that needn't be refrigerated until they are opened. They are available in tasty flavors such as chocolate, mocha, and vanilla. You can substitute mashed tofu in recipes that call for ricotta or cottage cheese. Although soy cheeses are often recommended to the cheese lover, be aware that this alternative product may contain casein, a cow's milk protein. The protein is added to soy cheese to give it the "stretchy" consistency as it melts. Even ice cream and other yummy frozen desserts are available made from soy beans, rice, and fruit.

3. Eliminate or reduce your intake of eggs.

By eliminating eggs, you will eliminate one of the most concentrated sources of cholesterol in the diet. At first, you may wish to limit your use of eggs to no more than three a week. Try removing at least one egg yolk, as this is the primary source of cholesterol and saturated fat. In place of scrambled eggs in the morning, you may opt to try some of the egg-replacement products available. Better yet, try scrambled tofu in place of eggs for breakfast.

4. Eliminate or reduce refined flours, grains, and sugars.

By eliminating refined sugars from your diet, you will enjoy a restored balance in energy and lose the terrible cravings that are associated with a diet high in refined sugars. In place of refined sugar you may wish to try barley malt syrup, brown rice syrup, and date sugar. These sweeteners can be found at most natural foods markets. In place of sweets, rely on fresh fruit. By choosing brown rice over polished white rice you will enjoy a richer source of vitamins, minerals, and natural bran, as well as a more hearty flavor. The same benefits come from choosing whole-wheat flour over refined white flour. Choose whole-wheat breads, rolls, muffins, and tortillas, too.

5. Eliminate or reduce butter, margarine, mayonnaise, and oils.

Butter, margarine, and mayonnaise, what I call "luxury fats," are rich in saturated fat, dangerous trans-fats, and cholesterol. It is important that you cut back on your consumption of these foods. Soon you will really begin to taste the breads you may have previously smothered in butter. In place of butter and margarine, try apple butter, non-sugared fruit spreads, and nut butters.

Limit your use of vegetable oils. Refer to the section on fats and oils in Chapter Six for the proper purchase, care, and use of oils. In place of oil, use vegetable stock to cook and sauté vegetables and in the preparation of other dishes.

6. Increase your intake of fresh, organic vegetables and fruits.

For their abundance of fiber and density of antioxidant vitamins, minerals, and cancer-fighting phytochemicals, choose fresh vegetables and fruits more often. For variety, include new fruits and vegetables you haven't tried. Have fruit salad for breakfast, make fruit smoothies, and carry fruit with you as an "anytime snack." Try to consume most of your fruit whole rather than juiced. Whole fruit retains its important fiber, and its natural sugars are assimilated more slowly. As juice, fruit sugars can be assimilated too quickly. You can dilute the concentration of juices by "halving" them with water.

Use vegetables in pasta, steamed, over rice, or in a marinara. Cut up vegetables and fruit in advance to keep them handy as a snack throughout the day, and store washed and cut fruits and vegetables in the fridge to make your next meal preparation quick and easy.

You will probably find that after about a month of following the Revised American Diet, you will have successfully overcome the urge to slip backwards and consume unhealthy animal products as well as foods high in sodium and refined sugars. After only two weeks, you will have naturally lost unwanted body weight, show markedly better-looking skin, and feel more energized throughout the day. You may notice that symptoms like chronic congestion, persistent headaches, gas, and indigestion seem to vanish. You will probably find that you need less sleep and wake up feeling rejuvenated rather than sluggish. If you have been taking medications, you may find that they are no longer necessary (although always check with your physician before making such changes). If you have your cholesterol and blood pressure checked prior to making the transition and then again in two months, you will likely see a continuing decrease in both.

Remember, by following the guidelines suggested in this chapter, you will dramatically reduce your cholesterol level, blood pressure, body fat, and your risk of developing heart attack, stroke, cancer, hypertension, diabetes, obesity, osteoporosis, and dental disease.

DINING OUT

Eating at restaurants as a vegetarian is much easier than you might think. These days there is a heightened awareness of different eating concerns, and restaurants are not only willing to be accommodating, but some specifically cater to vegetarians.

In almost any restaurant, you should have no problem asking for a plate of steamed vegetables and rice. You can also always order a meal-sized salad and request that dressings be served on the side. In place of dressing, ask for a few lemon wedges to squeeze over your greens. Better yet, bring your own favorite dressing with you. Many restaurants also offer full salad bars where you can find an abundance of vegetables such as broccoli, cucumbers, onions, celery, peppers, tomatoes, carrots, and sprouts. Be careful when choosing a dressing from these bars, however. Most often they serve commercial dressings that not only contain eggs and milk products, but are also extremely high in both sodium and sugar.

Italian restaurants have an abundance of pasta dishes from which to choose. If you see one you'd like that is prepared with a cream sauce, simply ask your waiter to substitute a marinara or classic red sauce. Polenta, a coarse cornmeal, is also often found on the menus of Italian restaurants, usually served with a marinara or vegetable sauce. Another common dish is risotto (rice), often made with saffron and mixed vegetables.

Chinese restaurants can be another haven for vegetarian diners. Many of their dishes are centered on vegetables and rice. You will also find tofu dishes. Unfortunately, some Chinese restaurants continue to use MSG as a seasoning. Not only is this a source of sodium, but some people have allergic reactions to it. Also, salt and oil are often used liberally in the preparation of Chinese dishes. Ask your waiter if your dish can be prepared without these three items.

At **Mexican restaurants** you can always ask for a hearty vegetarian burrito made from rice, beans, salsa, and vegetables. Be sure to request that they hold the cheese, since it is often automatically added to burritos. Ask your waitperson if the restaurant uses lard or oils in the preparation of their beans. Neither of these will be a healthy addition to what is otherwise a nutritious meal.

At **Middle Eastern restaurants** you can choose from a variety of vegetable, grain, and legume dishes. A popular dish is Yalanji Yaprak, which is baked eggplant stuffed with vegetables. Another healthful dish is couscous, which is steamed bulgur wheat, served with vegetables.

Even in the worst situations you usually have a choice. Most chefs are happy to prepare a plate of rice and vegetables for their vegan customers. Many of today's fast-food establishments are providing hearty baked potatoes stuffed with broccoli or cauliflower and offer salad bars to complement the meal.

If you have been invited to eat at a friend's house, let your host or hostess know that you are a vegetarian so they have time to prepare for you. Some people have told me that it makes them uncomfortable, thinking that explaining that they are vegetarian is demanding or rude. On the contrary, I have found that people would much rather know what my preferences are in advance and try to accommodate them rather than see me avoiding their food later. You can always offer to bring your favorite dish. If you are not yet comfortable with your new vegetarian lifestyle and/or believe that your host might be hurt by your desire not to eat certain foods, you can always say that you are under the strict orders of your doctor.

CHAPTER FOURTEEN

RECIPES AND COOKING GUIDES

You can say no to any food offered you by any person on this planet.
If that person is offended, there's a problem, but the problem isn't yours.
—Victoria Moran

To help you make the transition to healthy and wholesome eating, four talented chefs have contributed a total of thirty-seven delicious vegetarian recipes to this chapter, including soups, salads, pastas, tofu burgers, corn bread, and even pancakes. The recipe section is followed by helpful guides for cooking a variety of grains and legumes, as well as suggestions for tasty vegetable and seasoning combinations.

JENNIFER RAYMOND

Jennifer Raymond has a Master's degree in nutrition and is a popular cooking and nutrition instructor throughout the United States. She works as a chef and dietitian with Dean Ornish, M.D., in his "Open Your Heart" program, teaching patients how a delicious, easily prepared vegetarian diet can reverse heart disease. Her first cookbook, *The Best of Jenny's Kitchen*, was published by Avon books in 1981 and was followed by her television series *Cooking–Naturally!* In 1992, she published *The Peaceful Palate*.

WHOLE-WHEAT PANCAKES

Makes 12 3-inch pancakes

These pancakes are simple to prepare and delicious with fresh fruit or fresh fruit preserves.

INGREDIENTS

1 cup whole wheat flour
$\frac{1}{2}$ teaspoon baking powder
$\frac{1}{4}$ teaspoon baking soda
$\frac{1}{4}$ teaspoon salt
1 $\frac{1}{2}$ cups soy milk or rice milk
1 tablespoon maple syrup
1 tablespoon vinegar

Stir the flour, baking powder, baking soda, and salt together in a mixing bowl. Add the soy or rice milk, maple syrup, and vinegar. Stir just enough to remove any lumps.

Preheat an oil-sprayed or nonstick skillet or griddle. Pour small amounts of batter onto the heated surface and cook until the tops bubble. Turn with a spatula and cook the second side until golden brown. Serve immediately.

CORNBREAD

Makes 9 3x3 inch pieces

Be sure to try this quick-to-mix cornbread made without eggs.

INGREDIENTS

1 $\frac{1}{2}$ cups soy milk
1 $\frac{1}{2}$ tablespoon vinegar
1 cup cornmeal
1 cup flour (unbleached or whole wheat pastry)
2 tablespoons sugar or other sweetener
1 teaspoon baking powder
$\frac{1}{2}$ teaspoon baking soda
$\frac{3}{4}$ teaspoon salt
2 tablespoons oil

Preheat the oven to 425°F.

Combine the soy milk and vinegar and set aside. Mix the cornmeal, flour, sugar, baking powder, baking soda and salt in a large bowl. Add the soy milk mixture and the oil. Stir until just blended. Spread the batter into a nonstick or lightly oil-sprayed 9 x 9-inch baking dish, and bake for 25 to 30 minutes. Serve hot.

COUSCOUS SALAD

Serves 6

Couscous is the world's smallest pasta. It cooks almost instantly and makes a colorful and flavorful salad.

INGREDIENTS

1 cup couscous
1 cup boiling water
$\frac{1}{2}$ small red onion, finely chopped
1 red bell pepper, diced
1 carrot, grated
$\frac{1}{2}$ cup finely shredded red cabbage
$\frac{1}{2}$ cup green peas, fresh or frozen
$\frac{1}{2}$ cup currants or raisins
1 tablespoon balsamic vinegar
2 tablespoons seasoned rice vinegar
1 teaspoon toasted sesame oil
1 teaspoon low-sodium soy sauce
1 teaspoon Dijon mustard
1 teaspoon curry powder

Place the couscous in a large bowl and pour the boiling water over it. Stir to mix, then cover and let stand until cooled. Fluff with a fork.

When the couscous is cool, add the onion, bell pepper, carrot, cabbage, peas, and currants or raisins.

To make the dressing, mix the vinegars, sesame oil, soy sauce, mustard and curry powder. Pour over the salad and toss to mix.

MOCK TUNA SALAD

Makes 4 sandwiches

This spread is delicious and easy to prepare, and you don't risk the mercury and other contaminants often found in tunafish.

INGREDIENTS

1 15-ounce can garbanzo beans, drained
1 stalk celery, finely chopped
1 carrot, grated (optional)
1 green onion, finely chopped
2 teaspoons eggless mayonnaise
1 tablespoon sweet pickle relish
$\frac{1}{4}$ teaspoon salt (optional)

Mash the garbanzo beans with a fork or potato masher. Leave some chunks. Add the sliced celery, grated carrot, chopped onion, mayonnaise and relish. Add salt to taste. Serve on whole wheat bread or pita bread with lettuce and sliced tomatoes.

For a fat-free version substitute 2 teaspoons of mustard for the 2 teaspoons of mayonnaise.

QUICK CHILI

Serves 8

There's nothing quite like a bowl of steaming hot chili to warm a cold winter day. Textured vegetable protein adds flavor and texture and is available in natural food stores.

INGREDIENTS

1 onion, chopped
1 green bell pepper, diced
2 large garlic cloves, minced
2 15-ounce cans pinto beans
1 15-ounce can tomato sauce
1 cup corn, fresh or frozen
$\frac{1}{2}$ cup textured vegetable protein
1-2 teaspoons chili powder
1 teaspoon oregano
$\frac{1}{2}$ teaspoon ground cumin
$\frac{1}{8}$ teaspoon cayenne (more for spicier beans)

Heat ½ cup of water in a large pot, then add the onion, bell pepper, and garlic. Cook over high heat, stirring often, until the onion is soft, about 5 minutes. Add an additional ½ cup of water and all the remaining ingredients. Simmer at least 30 minutes.

TOFU BURGERS

Makes 8 burgers

These burgers are quick and easy to make. The ingredients can be mixed in advance and stored in the refrigerator for up to a week. Form and cook the patties as needed. Or you can cook all the patties at one time, then store them in the refrigerator and reheat them in a toaster oven or microwave. If you want to grill the burgers, precook the patties before putting them on the grill.

INGREDIENTS

1 lb. firm tofu, mashed
½ cup quick-cooking rolled oats
1 slice whole wheat bread, finely crumbled
1 small onion, finely chopped, or 2 tablespoons onion powder
1 ½ tablespoons finely chopped parsley
3 tablespoons soy sauce
1 teaspoon garlic powder
½ teaspoon each: basil, oregano, cumin
8 whole wheat burger buns
8 lettuce leaves
8 tomato slices
8 red onion slices
eggless mayonnaise, mustard, ketchup, barbecue sauce, etc.

Mix the tofu with the rolled oats, bread crumbs, chopped onion, parsley, soy sauce and seasonings. Knead for a minute or so, until the mixture holds together. Shape into 8 patties. Lightly spray a large skillet (preferably nonstick) with oil, then cook the patties on both sides until golden brown. Toast the buns, garnish them with all your favorite trimmings, then top each off with a tofu patty.

Baked version: Place the tofu patties on oil-sprayed baking sheet. Bake at 350°F until lightly browned, about 25 minutes.

MIDDLE EASTERN LENTILS AND RICE

Serves 8

This is a popular dish in the Middle East. Traditionally, the lentil and rice mixture is topped with green salad and lemon vinaigrette. The combination of the peppery lentils with the cool salad and tart vinaigrette is marvelous.

INGREDIENTS

1 tablespoon olive oil
2 large onions, coarsely chopped
$\frac{3}{4}$ cups brown rice
$1\frac{1}{2}$ teaspoon salt
$1\frac{1}{2}$ cups lentils, rinsed
4 cups boiling water
4-6 cups leaf lettuce or salad mix
1-2 tomatoes
2-3 green onions
1 cucumber, thinly sliced
1 avocado, sliced
2 tablespoons olive oil
2 tablespoons lemon juice
1 teaspoon sugar or other sweetener
$\frac{1}{2}$ teaspoon paprika
$\frac{1}{4}$ teaspoon dry mustard
1 garlic clove, pressed
$\frac{1}{4}$ teaspoon salt

Heat 1 tablespoon of olive oil in a large pot and sauté the onions until soft, about 5 minutes. Add the rice and $1\frac{1}{2}$ teaspoons of salt. Cook for 3 minutes. Stir in the lentils and boiling water. Bring to a simmer, then cover and cook until the rice and lentils are tender, about 50 minutes.

While the lentil mixture is cooking, prepare a generous green salad using leaf lettuce or salad mix, tomatoes, green onions, cucumber and avocado. Feel free to add any other ingredients you'd enjoy in the salad.

Combine the remaining olive oil with the lemon juice, sugar, paprika, dry mustard, garlic and salt. Mix well then pour over the salad. Toss to mix.

To serve, place a portion of the lentil mixture on each plate and top with a generous serving of salad.

MEXICAN CORN PIE

Serves 8 to 10

Serve this spicy rice and corn pie with Quick Chili (see p.183) and a crisp green salad.

INGREDIENTS

1 cup brown basmati rice (or other long-grain rice)
1 large onion, chopped
2 large garlic cloves, crushed
1 red bell pepper, diced
2 cups fresh or frozen corn
1 4-ounce can diced chilies
1 cup oatmeal
1 teaspoon salt
1 teaspoon cumin
2 tablespoons nutritional yeast (optional)
3 cups soy milk or rice milk

Bring 4 cups of water to a boil and add the rice. Bring to a slow boil, then cover, and cook until rice is tender, about 40 minutes. Pour off excess liquid.

In a large oven-proof skillet, heat $\frac{1}{2}$ cup water and cook the onion, garlic, and bell pepper until the onion is soft, about 5 minutes. Remove from the heat and stir in all the remaining ingredients, including the cooked rice.

Bake at 350°F for 45 minutes.

SOYOUNG MACK

Tiger Rose Fine Foods

SoYoung Mack is the owner and executive chef of Tiger Rose Fine Foods, a gourmet carry-out shop and catering business in Mill Valley, California. Her approach to cooking is intuitive, and guided by the seasons. Her goal in preparing foods is to bring customers healthful food of the highest quality, well balanced in seasonings, textures, and colors, very pleasing in both taste and appearance. These recipes are a sampling of some of her most popular vegan salads.

THAI VEGETABLE SLAW

Makes approximately 8 cups

INGREDIENTS

$1\frac{1}{2}$ cups sliced red cabbage ($2\frac{1}{2}$" x $\frac{1}{8}$" strips)
$1\frac{1}{2}$ cups sliced green cabbage ($2\frac{1}{2}$" x $\frac{1}{8}$" strips)
$\frac{1}{2}$ cup julienned sweet peppers ($2\frac{1}{2}$" x $\frac{1}{8}$" strips)
$1\frac{1}{2}$ cups julienned carrots ($2\frac{1}{2}$" x $\frac{1}{8}$" strips)
1 cup lightly blanched snap or snow peas
1 cup lightly blanched broccoli florets
$\frac{1}{2}$ cup peanuts
3 tablespoons chopped cilantro

Toss all ingredients in a bowl with $\frac{1}{2}$ cup Chile-Lime Dressing (on the following page) or to taste.

THAI CHILE-LIME DRESSING

Makes approximately 2 cups

INGREDIENTS

1 ½ cups lime juice
½ cup unseasoned rice vinegar
2 tablespoons Thai fish sauce (substitute 2 tablespoons low-sodium
    soy sauce for vegan version)
4 tablespoons soy sauce
6 tablespoons barley malt syrup
½ teaspoon ground cumin
1 tablespoon crushed garlic
6 tablespoons grated ginger
½ teaspoon Indonesian sambal (substitute Tabasco if not available)

JAPANESE CUCUMBER SALAD

Makes approximately 4 cups

INGREDIENTS

3 cups English cucumbers, stripe-peeled and
    sliced into ½ moons, ⅛" thick
¾ cup julienne carrots, 2 ½" x ¹/₁₆" x ¹/₁₆"
¼ cup julienne sweet red pepper, 2 ½" x ¹/₁₆" x ¹/₁₆"
1 tablespoon toasted, hulled sesame seeds

Toss all ingredients in a bowl with ½ cup Japanese Cucumber Marinade (following)
or to taste.

JAPANESE CUCUMBER MARINADE

Makes approximately 1³/₄ cups

INGREDIENTS

1 cup unseasoned rice vinegar
¹/₃ cup apple cider vinegar
2 tablespoons + 1 teaspoon water
2 tablespoons + 1 teaspoon fructose crystals
2¹/₂ teaspoons grated ginger

Place all ingredients into a stainless-steel saucepan. Heat at medium-low for 2-3 minutes until sugar has dissolved. Cool at least 10 minutes before pouring over vegetables.

QUINOA OR BULGUR WHEAT SALAD

Makes approximately 10 cups

INGREDIENTS

2³/₄ cups water
1 teaspoon Madras curry powder
¹/₈ teaspoon ground turmeric
¹/₈ teaspoon ground cardamom
¹/₈ teaspoon ground cloves
²/₃ teaspoon salt
1 teaspoon crushed garlic
2 cups quinoa or bulgur wheat
   (quinoa must be rinsed with cold water and drained in
   a fine sieve; bulgur requires no special preparation)
1 cup diced tomatoes
1 cup fresh corn, lightly sautéed in olive oil or steamed
1 cup cauliflower florets, lightly blanched
¹/₂ cup fresh or frozen English peas, lightly blanched

Bring water and spices to a boil in a 2-quart saucepan. Lower heat and add the quinoa or bulgur. Cover the pot with a tightly fitted lid and simmer at low heat for 15 minutes. Transfer the quinoa or bulgur into a 3-quart salad bowl and allow it to cool for 30 minutes. Add the vegetables and Honey-Curry Dressing (below) to taste.

HONEY-CURRY DRESSING

Makes approximately 3 cups

INGREDIENTS

1 tablespoon grated ginger
1 tablespoon Dijon mustard
9 tablespoons honey
1 cup apple cider vinegar
1 cup peanut oil
$1\frac{1}{2}$ tablespoons Madras curry
$\frac{1}{4}$ teaspoon ground cinnamon
$\frac{1}{8}$ teaspoon ground clove
$\frac{1}{4}$ teaspoon ground black pepper
$\frac{1}{4}$ teaspoon salt

BEET SALAD

Makes approximately 4 $\frac{1}{2}$ cups

INGREDIENTS

3 cups cooked julienned (cut into strips), beets, 1 $\frac{1}{2}$" x $\frac{1}{4}$" x $\frac{1}{4}$"
$\frac{1}{2}$ cup julienned carrots, 1 $\frac{1}{2}$" x $\frac{1}{16}$" x $\frac{1}{16}$"
$\frac{1}{2}$ cup green apples, peeled and sliced into thin wedges
$\frac{1}{4}$ cup toasted walnuts, coarsely chopped

To prepare the beets: Boil 4-6 medium beets until a knife easily pierces the flesh to the core. Rinse with cold water and push the skin off the beets with your hands (you might want to wear rubber gloves to avoid staining your hands). Trim the ends of unwanted fibers. Cut into julienned sticks, 1 $\frac{1}{2}$" x $\frac{1}{4}$" x $\frac{1}{4}$". Toss with all remaining ingredients in a bowl with $\frac{1}{4}$ cup Balsamic Vinaigrette (following) or to taste.

BALSAMIC VINAIGRETTE FOR BEETS

Makes approximately 2 $\frac{3}{4}$ cups

INGREDIENTS

3 tablespoons Dijon mustard
$\frac{1}{2}$ cup honey
1 cup balsamic vinegar
1 cup walnut oil
$\frac{1}{4}$ teaspoon salt
$\frac{1}{8}$ teaspoon ground black pepper

Mix all ingredients together in a jar or cruet and store, tightly covered, in the refrigerator.

KEITH A. LORD
Lark Creek Inn

Award-winning chef Keith A. Lord is a graduate of the New England Culinary Institute in Essex, Vermont. A native of California, he has practiced his culinary craft throughout New England, in Virginia, Los Angeles, San Francisco, and the Hawaiian Islands. He is currently the sous-chef at the historic Lark Creek Inn in Larkspur, California.

ROASTED VEGETABLE SANDWICH
Makes 4 servings

INGREDIENTS

1 eggplant, cut in $\frac{1}{4}$" thick slices
1 yellow bell pepper, seeded and cut into 4 pieces
1 red bell pepper, seeded and cut into 4 pieces
2 zucchinis, each cut into 4 slices
1 red onion, cut into $\frac{1}{4}$" thick slices
1 tablespoon garlic, sliced
2 tablespoons olive oil
salt and pepper to taste
1 tablespoon fresh marjoram
Sandwich bread, pita, or focaccia

Preheat oven to 375°F. Brush all the vegetables and garlic lightly with the olive oil. Place the vegetables on a baking tray. Sprinkle with salt, pepper, and marjoram. Roast for 35-45 minutes until slightly soft and a bit browned. Serve on sandwich bread, pita, or focaccia.

TOFU SCRAMBLE

Makes 4 servings

INGREDIENTS

2 tablespoons virgin olive oil
1 onion, sliced thin
1 green bell pepper, cut into $\frac{1}{2}$" squares
1 red bell pepper, cut into $\frac{1}{2}$" squares
$\frac{1}{2}$ lb. tofu, cut into $\frac{1}{2}$" squares
$\frac{1}{2}$ cup mushrooms, sliced
$\frac{1}{2}$ cup asparagus, cut into $\frac{1}{2}$" pieces
1 ripe tomato, cut into $\frac{1}{2}$" pieces
$\frac{1}{2}$ teaspoon dried thyme
$\frac{1}{4}$ teaspoon cayenne pepper
1 tablespoon parsley, chopped
salt and freshly ground pepper to taste

Place the oil in a skillet over medium heat. Add the onion and sauté for 2 minutes. Add the peppers, sauté for 2 additional minutes. Add the remaining ingredients and heat through. Serve immediately.

GRAIN PILAF

Makes 4-6 servings

INGREDIENTS

1 cup bulgur
1 cup couscous
1 cup lentils
$\frac{1}{4}$ cup sundried tomatoes, soaked in warm water, chopped
1 tablespoon olives, finely chopped
$\frac{1}{2}$ bunch parsley
salt and freshly ground pepper to taste

To make the bulgur: Cover the bulgur with $1\frac{1}{2}$ cups boiling water. Mix well, cover and let stand 30 minutes. In a strainer squeeze all remaining liquid from the bulgur. To make the couscous: Cover with $1\frac{1}{2}$ cups boiling water. Mix well, cover, and let stand 10 minutes. Add 2 tablespoons virgin olive oil and mix in gently.

To make the lentils: Cover with 3 cups water, bring to a boil. Reduce to a simmer and cook until tender, 15-20 minutes. Drain.

In a large bowl, combine the bulgur, couscous and lentils with all the remaining ingredients, season with salt and pepper. Serve.

SWEET VEGETABLE RISOTTO

Makes 4 to 6 servings

INGREDIENTS

3 cups carrot juice
3 cups celery juice
$\frac{1}{4}$ cup virgin olive oil
$\frac{1}{2}$ teaspoon garlic, minced
1 $\frac{3}{4}$ cups arborio rice
$\frac{1}{2}$ cup chardonnay
$\frac{1}{2}$ cup carrots, split and sliced
$\frac{1}{2}$ cup green beans, cut in 1–inch pieces
$\frac{1}{2}$ cup zucchini, split and sliced
$\frac{1}{2}$ cup asparagus, cut in $\frac{1}{2}$ inch pieces
$\frac{1}{2}$ cup red bell pepper, seeded and sliced
$\frac{1}{2}$ cup freshly shelled peas
$\frac{1}{3}$ cup scallions, sliced
1 teaspoon kosher salt
$\frac{1}{2}$ teaspoon freshly ground black pepper
1 tablespoon flat leaf parsley, chopped

Bring the carrot and celery juices to a simmer in a saucepan. In a 4-quart skillet, heat the olive oil over medium heat. Add the garlic and rice and stir until coated with oil. Add the wine and bring to a boil. When the wine is absorbed, add the carrots and green beans. Pour $\frac{1}{2}$ cup of the simmering juice mixture into the rice pan; stir until it is absorbed. Continue adding the juice until three-quarters of it has been used, about 15-20 minutes. Add the remaining vegetables. Continue ladling and stirring in the remaining juice about 10 minutes more, until the rice is al dente. Season with salt and pepper and top with parsley.

ORANGE MASHED SWEET POTATOES

Makes 4 servings

INGREDIENTS

2 lbs. sweet potatoes, cut into large dice
4 oz. fresh orange juice
salt and freshly ground pepper to taste

In a large pot, boil the potatoes until soft, drain, and let stand in a strainer for 5 minutes. Mash the potatoes in a large bowl and add the orange juice, salt, and pepper. Stir to combine.

TABBOULEH

Makes 6 servings

INGREDIENTS

$\frac{1}{2}$ cup bulgur
$\frac{1}{2}$ cup green onions, finely chopped
1 cup parsley
$\frac{1}{2}$ cup mint, finely chopped
2 cups tomatoes, coarsely chopped
$\frac{1}{3}$ cup lemon juice
$\frac{1}{2}$ teaspoon salt
$\frac{1}{4}$ teaspoon pepper
$\frac{1}{2}$ tablespoon virgin olive oil

Soak the bulgur in cold water and cover for 10 minutes. Drain and squeeze as dry as possible in a towel or strainer. Add all the remaining ingredients except for the oil; combine and let stand for 30 minutes. Stir in the olive oil.

CHILEAN VEGETABLE STEW

Makes 4 servings

INGREDIENTS

1 ½ cups cranberry beans, dried
1 onion, roughly chopped
4 tablespoons canola oil
1 garlic clove, minced
6 tomatoes, roughly chopped
½ teaspoon dried basil
1 ½ teaspoons dried oregano
½ teaspoon dried thyme
salt and freshly ground pepper to taste
2 cups winter squash, peeled, cut into large dice
⅓ cup corn kernels

In a medium saucepan, cover the beans with cold water and bring to a boil. Remove from heat and soak for 1 hour. Change the water, bring to a boil, and reduce to a simmer for 1 hour. In a large skillet, slow cook the onion in the oil until soft, then add the garlic, tomatoes, basil, oregano, thyme, salt, and pepper. Cook over low heat until mixture is thick. Add the squash and beans. Cook until the beans are completely done. Stir in the corn and cook until heated through. Serve with pebre.

PEBRE

Makes 2 cups

INGREDIENTS

2 tablespoons canola oil
1 tablespoon lemon juice
½ cup water
½ cup cilantro, finely chopped
1 garlic clove, finely chopped
½ teaspoon salt
4 habanero chilies, seeded and finely chopped

Combine all ingredients and refrigerate.

SOUTHWESTERN CORN AND BLACK BEAN SALSA

Makes 1 quart

INGREDIENTS

$\frac{1}{2}$ pint black beans
2 ears corn, or 1 $\frac{1}{4}$ cups kernels
2 tomatoes, medium diced
1 jalapeño, seeded and finely diced
3 cloves garlic, finely chopped
1 red onion, finely diced
2 oz. red wine vinegar
1 teaspoon dried oregano
1 teaspoon cumin, ground
$\frac{1}{2}$ bunch cilantro, rinsed, picked, and roughly chopped
salt and freshly ground pepper to taste

Prepare and combine all the ingredients.

GARLIC VINAIGRETTE DRESSING

Makes 3 cups

INGREDIENTS

1 cup tomato sauce
$\frac{2}{3}$ cup tomato juice
4 tablespoons parsley, chopped
4 tablespoons red wine vinegar
4 tablespoons fresh-squeezed lemon juice
2 tablespoons virgin olive oil
2 tablespoons Dijon mustard
6 cloves garlic, finely chopped

Combine all the ingredients and whisk together. Cover tightly. Refrigerate for 24 hours.

CUBAN–STYLE BLACK BEANS

Makes 4 servings

INGREDIENTS

1 lb. black beans
2 onions
2 green bell peppers
2 tablespoons virgin olive oil
3 cloves garlic, finely chopped
$\frac{1}{2}$ teaspoon cumin, ground
1 bay leaf
$\frac{1}{2}$ cup tomato sauce
salt to taste
1 tablespoon sherry wine vinegar

Wash the beans and soak them, covered, overnight. Split 1 onion and 1 bell pepper (seeds removed) in half, and add to the beans. Bring the beans to a boil, then simmer for 1$\frac{1}{2}$ hours. Heat the oil in a pan and sauté the remaining onion, pepper, and the garlic until the onion is translucent. Add the cumin, bay leaf, and tomato sauce and cook for 5 minutes. Remove the bay leaf and blend the mixture in a blender. Add to the beans, season with salt. Discard the onion and pepper halves and add the vinegar.

LEMON AND PEPPER RICE PILAF

Makes 4 servings

INGREDIENTS

1 onion, finely diced
2 tablespoons virgin olive oil
1 clove garlic, finely minced
Zest of 2 lemons
2 cups basmati rice
3 cups vegetable stock
1 teaspoon salt
$\frac{1}{2}$ tablespoon cracked pepper

In a heavy-bottomed saucepan sauté the onion in the oil over low heat until translucent. Add the garlic and lemon zest and cook for 4 minutes. Add rice, stir well. Add the stock and salt. Bring to a simmer, cover and cook over low heat for 18 minutes. Open the pan and add the pepper, cover and cook for 3 minutes longer. Remove from heat and let stand, covered, for 2 minutes. Season with more salt and pepper if desired.

TOFU CREOLE

Makes 6 servings

INGREDIENTS

4 tablespoons virgin olive oil
$\frac{1}{3}$ cup whole-wheat flour
$\frac{3}{4}$ cup onion, diced
$\frac{1}{2}$ cup celery, diced
$\frac{1}{2}$ cup bell pepper, seeded and diced
1 14-oz. can tomato sauce
1 $\frac{1}{2}$ lbs. tofu, cut into 1" squares
1 $\frac{3}{4}$ cups hot water
$\frac{1}{2}$ teaspoon dried thyme
1 bay leaf
2 teaspoons honey
1 clove garlic, finely chopped
salt and freshly ground pepper to taste
2 tablespoons parsley, chopped

In a large skillet heat the oil, add the flour, and brown lightly. Add the onion, celery, and bell pepper and sauté for 3 minutes. Add the tomato sauce, tofu, water, thyme, bay leaf, honey, garlic, and salt and pepper. Stir well, cover, and simmer for 20 minutes, stirring occasionally. Add the parsley before serving. Serve over brown rice.

RIGATONI WITH FRESH TOMATOES

Makes 4 servings

INGREDIENTS

1 lb. pasta
1 onion, diced
4 cups tomatoes, roughly chopped
2 cloves garlic, finely chopped
salt to taste
$\frac{1}{2}$ tablespoon honey
$\frac{1}{4}$ cup parsley, fresh, chopped
$\frac{1}{4}$ cup basil, fresh, chopped
$\frac{1}{4}$ cup sage, fresh, chopped
$\frac{1}{4}$ cup oregano, fresh, chopped
$\frac{1}{4}$ cup sorrel, fresh, chopped

Bring water to a boil and cook the pasta. While the pasta is cooking, sauté the onion in the oil until it starts to brown. Add the tomatoes and garlic, bring to a boil. Reduce the heat to medium and let cook 5 minutes. Add the salt, honey, and herbs. Toss with the cooked rigatoni pasta, serve.

ANNIE SOMERVILLE

Greens Restaurant

Annie Somerville is the executive chef at Greens in San Francisco, and the author of *Fields of Greens*, published by Bantam Dell Doubleday. Greens, a culinary landmark since 1982, is credited with bringing vegetarian cooking to the forefront. Working closely with nearby Green Gulch Farm, the staff at Greens prides itself in being able to include locally grown, garden-fresh organic produce in dishes centered around pasta, dried beans, and grains.

VEGETABLE STOCK

Makes about 7 cups

INGREDIENTS

1 yellow onion, thinly sliced
1 leek top, washed and chopped
4 garlic cloves, in their skin, crushed with the side of a knife blade
1 teaspoon salt
2 medium carrots, chopped
1 large potato, thinly sliced
$\frac{1}{4}$ lb. white mushrooms, sliced
2 celery ribs, sliced
6 parsley sprigs, coarsely chopped
6 fresh thyme sprigs
2 fresh marjoram or oregano sprigs
3 fresh sage leaves
2 bay leaves
$\frac{1}{2}$ teaspoon peppercorns
9 cups cold water

Pour just enough water into a stockpot to start the onion cooking. Add the onion, leek top, garlic, and salt. Stir the vegetables, then cover the pot, and cook them gently over medium heat for 15 minutes. Add the remaining ingredients and cover with 9 cups cold water. Bring to a boil, reduce the heat, and simmer, uncovered, for 1 hour. Pour the stock through a strainer, pressing as much liquid as possible from the vegetables, then discard them.

Variation: Light Vegetable Stock: Lighter in flavor and color, this stock goes into potato soups to keep them from discoloring. Using the main recipe, add an extra potato, omit the carrots and mushrooms, and use the entire leek. The tops and outer leaves of fennel bulbs are excellent additions.

SUMMER MINESTRONE

Makes 8 to 9 cups

INGREDIENTS

$\frac{1}{2}$ cup dried red beans, about 3 oz., sorted and soaked overnight
6 cups cold water
2 bay leaves
2 fresh sage leaves
1 fresh oregano sprig
1 tablespoon extra virgin olive oil
1 medium–size red onion, diced, about 2 cups
1 $\frac{1}{2}$ teaspoon salt
$\frac{1}{8}$ teaspoon pepper
$\frac{1}{4}$ teaspoon dried basil
$\frac{1}{4}$ teaspoon dried oregano
6 garlic cloves, finely chopped
1 small carrot, diced, about $\frac{3}{4}$ cup
1 small red bell pepper, seeded and diced, about $\frac{3}{4}$ cup
1 small zucchini, diced, about $\frac{3}{4}$ cup
$\frac{1}{4}$ cup dry red wine
2 lbs. fresh tomatoes, peeled, seeded, and coarsely chopped, about 3 cups, or 1 28-oz. can tomatoes with juice, coarsely chopped
$\frac{1}{4}$ cup small elbow pasta, cooked al dente, drained, and rinsed
$\frac{1}{3}$ bunch of fresh spinach or chard, cut into thin ribbons and washed, about 2 cups packed
2 tablespoons chopped fresh basil

Drain and rinse the beans. Place them in a 2-quart saucepan with the water, 1 bay leaf, the sage leaves, and the oregano. Bring to a boil, reduce the heat, and simmer, uncovered, until the beans are tender, about 30 minutes. Remove the herbs.

While the beans are cooking, heat the olive oil in a soup pot. Add the onion, $\frac{1}{2}$ teaspoon salt, a few pinches of pepper, and the dried herbs. Sauté over medium heat until the onion is soft, 5 to 7 minutes. Add the garlic, carrots, peppers, and zucchini and sauté for 7 to 8 minutes. Add the wine and cook for 1 or 2 minutes, until the pan is almost dry. Add the tomatoes, 1 teaspoon salt, $\frac{1}{8}$ teaspoon pepper, and the remaining bay leaf. Simmer for 15 minutes, then add the pasta, spinach or chard, and beans with their broth. Season with salt and pepper to taste. Add the fresh basil just before serving.

TOMATO, SAFFRON, AND ROASTED GARLIC SOUP

Makes 8 to 9 cups

INGREDIENTS

Vegetable stock, about 5 cups; add 2 cups chopped canned tomatoes
1 head of garlic brushed with olive oil
2 lbs. fresh tomatoes, peeled and seeded or
  1 28-oz. can of tomatoes with juice
1 tablespoon extra virgin olive oil
1 medium-size yellow onion, diced, about 2 cups
$\frac{1}{4}$ teaspoon dried thyme
1 teaspoon salt and a pinch of pepper to taste
1 medium-size carrot, diced, about $\frac{3}{4}$ cup
1 celery rib, diced, about $\frac{1}{2}$ cup
1 medium-size yellow or red bell pepper, diced, about $\frac{3}{4}$ cup
5 garlic cloves, finely chopped
$\frac{1}{2}$ cup dry sherry
2 to 3 pinches saffron threads, to taste
1 bay leaf
3 tablespoons chopped Italian parsley

Make the stock (see page 199) and keep it warm over low heat.

Preheat the oven to 350°F. Place the whole head of garlic in a small baking dish, and roast for 30 minutes, until the cloves are very soft. When the garlic cools, cut the top off, squeeze the garlic out of its skin, and purée with the tomatoes in a blender or food processor.

Heat the olive oil in a sauté pan and add the onion, dried thyme, $\frac{1}{2}$ teaspoon salt, and a pinch of pepper. Sauté over medium heat for 5 minutes, then add the carrot, celery, peppers, and finely chopped garlic. Cook together until tender, then add the sherry and cook for 1 or 2 minutes, until the pan is almost dry. Add the tomato-garlic puree, the remaining $\frac{1}{2}$ teaspoon salt, a pinch of pepper, the saffron, bay leaf, and 4 to 5 cups stock. Cover and cook over low heat for at least 30 minutes. Add salt and pepper to taste. Garnish each serving with a sprinkle of Italian parsley.

SPICY BLACK BEAN SOUP

Makes 8 to 9 cups

INGREDIENTS

2 cups dried black beans, about 12 oz., sorted and soaked overnight
6 cups cold water
1 fresh oregano sprig
2 bay leaves
2 fresh sage leaves
1 tablespoon virgin olive oil
1 large yellow onion, thinly sliced, about 3 cups
1 $\frac{1}{2}$ teaspoons salt
$\frac{1}{8}$ teaspoon cayenne pepper
$\frac{1}{2}$ teaspoon dried oregano, toasted
8 garlic cloves, chopped
2 teaspoons Chipotle puree
1 heaped tablespoon Ancho chili puree
$\frac{1}{4}$ cup dry sherry
$\frac{1}{2}$ lb. fresh tomatoes, peeled, seeded, and chopped, about 1 cup, or
   1 8-oz. can tomatoes with juice, chopped
$\frac{1}{2}$ cup fresh orange juice
$\frac{1}{2}$ lb. fresh tomatoes, seeded and chopped, about 1 cup
1 tablespoon chopped cilantro

Rinse and drain the beans. Place them in a soup pot with the cold water, oregano, and bay and sage leaves. Bring to a boil, then reduce the heat and simmer, uncovered, until the beans are soft, 20 to 25 minutes.

Heat the olive oil in a sauté pan and add the onion, $\frac{1}{2}$ teaspoon of the salt, $\frac{1}{8}$ teaspoon cayenne, and the toasted oregano. Cook over medium heat until the onion is soft, 7 to 8 minutes. Add the garlic and the chili purées. Sauté for 3 to 4 minutes, add the sherry, and simmer until it is reduced by half, 1 or 2 minutes. Add the tomatoes and $\frac{1}{2}$ teaspoon of the salt and cook for 10 minutes.

Set aside 1 $\frac{1}{2}$ cups cooked beans and remove the fresh herbs and bay leaves. Combine the beans and their broth with the tomato and onion mixture and puree in a blender or food processor. Pass through a food mill to remove the bean skins and return the puree to the soup pot; add the reserved beans, the orange juice, and the $\frac{1}{2}$ teaspoon remaining salt. Season with salt and cayenne to taste. Cover and cook over low heat for 30 minutes.

Toss the tomatoes and cilantro together and garnish each serving with a spoonful.

MOROCCAN LENTIL SOUP

Makes 8 to 9 cups

INGREDIENTS

$\frac{3}{4}$ cup lentils, about 6 ounces
6 cups cold water
1 tablespoon extra virgin olive oil
1 medium-size yellow onion, diced, about 2 cups
1 teaspoon salt
Cayenne pepper to taste
1 small carrot, diced, about $\frac{1}{2}$ cup
1 celery rib, diced, about $\frac{1}{2}$ cup
1 small red or yellow bell pepper, seeded and diced, about $\frac{1}{2}$ cup
1 teaspoon cumin seed, toasted and ground
$\frac{1}{2}$ teaspoon ground coriander
$\frac{1}{8}$ teaspoon turmeric
4 garlic cloves, finely chopped
1 tablespoon grated fresh ginger
$\frac{1}{2}$ lb. fresh tomatoes, peeled, seeded, and chopped, about 1 cup, or
    1 8-oz. can tomatoes with juice, chopped
2 tablespoons chopped cilantro

Sort and rinse the lentils and place them in a soup pot with the cold water. Bring to a boil, then reduce the heat and simmer, uncovered, until tender, about 20 minutes.

While the lentils are cooking, heat the olive oil in a medium-size sauté pan and add the onion, $\frac{1}{2}$ teaspoon salt, and a few pinches of cayenne. Cook over medium heat until the onions are soft, 7 to 8 minutes, then add the vegetables, the other $\frac{1}{2}$ teaspoon salt, and the spices. Cook for 5 minutes, then stir in the garlic and ginger and cook for another minute or two. Add the vegetables and tomatoes to the lentils and their broth. Cover and cook for 30 minutes, allowing the flavors to blend and deepen. Season to taste with salt and cayenne. Garnish each serving with a sprinkle of cilantro.

CARROT SOUP WITH
NORTH AFRICAN SPICES

Makes 9 to 10 cups

INGREDIENTS

Light vegetable stock, about 5 cups; add 10 thin slices of ginger
1 tablespoon virgin olive oil
1 medium-size yellow onion, thinly sliced, about 1 ½ cups
1 ½ teaspoons salt
2 garlic cloves, finely chopped
1 ½ teaspoon cumin seed, toasted and ground
1 teaspoon coriander seed, toasted and ground
2 teaspoons grated fresh ginger
Cayenne pepper to taste
2 lbs. carrots, thinly sliced, about 7 cups
1 medium-size white potato or sweet potato, peeled and thinly
  sliced, about 1 cup
½ cup fresh orange juice
2 tablespoons coarsely chopped cilantro

Make the stock (see page 199) and keep it warm over low heat.

Heat the olive oil in a soup pot and add the onion and ½ teaspoon salt. Sauté over medium heat until it begins to release its juices, about 5 minutes, then add the garlic, cumin, coriander, ginger, and a few pinches of cayenne. Cook until the onion is very soft, about 10 minutes, adding a little stock if it sticks to the pan.

Add the carrots, the potato or sweet potato, 1 teaspoon salt, and 1 quart stock. Bring to a gentle boil, then reduce the heat, cover, and simmer until the carrots are very tender, about 15 minutes. Puree the soup in a blender or food processor until smooth, using a little extra stock if needed. Return to the pot, add the orange juice and more stock to the desired consistency. Season with salt to taste and, for additional heat, a pinch or two of cayenne. Garnish each serving with a sprinkle of cilantro.

COOKING BEANS

Soaking and cooking beans is much easier than most people believe. There are two approaches: the quick soak and the overnight soak.

QUICK SOAK

Prior to soaking, beans should be rinsed and picked over. Be sure to eliminate beans that are chipped or broken, as they are nutritionally inferior. Place beans in about three times their volume of hot water and bring to a boil. Boil for two minutes. Remove beans from heat and allow them to stand for one hour. Drain off the water and rinse the beans. Cover and cook for the times indicated in the recipes. Beans are done when they are easily mashed with a fork.

OVERNIGHT SOAK

After rinsing beans and eliminating those that are damaged, place beans in three times their volume of hot water. Allow to soak overnight, or at least four hours. The exception is soybeans, which require a full 12 hours of soaking. In the morning, drain water and rinse beans before cooking. Remember, lentils, split peas and black-eyed peas do not require soaking.

GRAIN (1/2 CUP)	COOKING TIMES FOR GRAINS		
	Water	Cooking Time	Yield (cups)
RICE (BROWN, LONG-GRAIN)	1 cup	30 minutes	1 $^1/_2$
RICE (BROWN, SHORT-GRAIN)	1 cup	40 minutes	1 $^1/_2$
RICE, BASMATI	$^1/_2$ cup	15 minutes	2
RICE, WILD	2 cups	50 minutes	2
RICE, WHITE	1 cup	20 minutes	1 $^3/_4$
WHOLE WHEAT BERRIES	1 $^1/_2$ cups	1 hour	1 $^1/_4$
BULGUR	1 cup	15 minutes	1 $^1/_2$
CRACKED WHEAT	1	15 minutes	1
RYE, BERRIES	1 $^1/_2$ cups	2 hours	1 $^1/_2$
RYE, FLAKES	1 $^1/_2$ cups	1 hour	1 $^1/_4$
OATS, ROLLED (QUICK)	1 cup	1 min. (stand 3 mins.)	1
OATS, OLD-FASHIONED	1 cup	5 minutes	1
BUCKWHEAT, GROATS	1 cup	15 minutes	1 $^3/_4$
BARLEY, FLAKES	1 $^1/_2$ cups	30 minutes	1
BARLEY, PEARL	1 $^1/_2$ cups	1 hour	2
CORNMEAL	2 cups	25 minutes	1 $^1/_2$ cups
QUINOA	1 cup	15 minutes	1 $^1/_4$ cups
MILLET	1 $^1/_3$ cups	40 minutes	2

LEGUME	COOKING TIMES FOR LEGUMES		
	Water	Cooking Time	Yield (cups)
ADZUKI BEANS (1/2 CUP)	2 cups	40 minutes	1 1/2
BLACK BEANS (1 CUP)	4 cups	2 hours	2
BLACK-EYED PEAS (1/2 CUP)	2 cups	1 hour	1 1/2
CHICKPEAS (1/2 CUP)	2 cups	1 hour	1 1/2
FAVA BEANS (1/2 CUP)	2 cups	40 minutes	1
GREAT NORTHERN BEANS (1/2 CUP)	2 cups	1 hour	1 1/2
KIDNEY BEANS (1/2 CUP)	2 cups	1 hour	1 1/2
LENTILS (1/2 CUP)	1 1/2 cups	40 minutes	1 1/2
LIMA BEANS (1 CUP)	2 cups	1 1/2 hours	1 1/4
MUNG BEANS (1 CUP)	2 1/2 cups	1 1/2 hours	2
NAVY BEANS (1 CUP)	3 cups	2 1/2 hours	2
PINTO BEANS (1/2 CUP)	2 cups	1 hour	1 1/2
RED BEANS (1 CUP)	3 cups	3 hours	2
SOYBEANS (1/2 CUP)	2 cups	2 hours, 20 min.	1 1/2
SPLIT PEAS (1/2 CUP)	2 cups	30 minutes	1

COMBINATIONS FOR ENJOYING VEGETABLES	
Corn and pimientos	Carrots and green beans
Cauliflower and green peas	Brussels sprouts and celery
Pearl onions, mushrooms, and green peas	Summer squash, tomatoes, and onions
Carrot slices and lima beans	Lima beans and corn
Mushrooms and green peas	Green cabbage, onions, and green bell pepper
Diced carrots and green beans	Brussels sprouts and carrot slices
Tomatoes, onions, and zucchini	Broccoli and cauliflower florets
Carrots, cabbage, and celery	Corn and peas
Celery and mushrooms	Eggplant, zucchini, onions, and tomatoes
Okra, onions, and tomatoes	

SEASONING COMBINATIONS FOR VEGETABLES	
In place of salt, there are a variety of seasonings to experiment with when preparing dishes. Below are a few combinations that work well with various vegetables and legumes.	
Beans (dried)	Basil, oregano, dill, savory, sage, cumin, garlic, parsley, bay leaf
Beans (green)	Basil, dill, marjoram, rosemary, thyme, oregano, savory
Beans (lima)	Basil, chives, marjoram, savory
Beets	Tarragon, dill, basil, thyme, bay leaf, cardamom seed
Broccoli	Tarragon, marjoram, oregano, basil
Brussels sprouts	Basil, dill, savory, caraway, thyme
Cabbage	Caraway, celery seed, savory, tarragon, dill, garlic
Carrots	Basil, dill, marjoram, thyme, coriander, parsley
Cauliflower	Basil, rosemary, savory, dill, tarragon
Eggplant	Basil, thyme, oregano, rosemary, sage, onion, garlic
Onions	Oregano, thyme, basil
Peas	Basil, mint, savory, oregano, dill
Potatoes	Dill, chives, basil, marjoram, savory, parsley
Spinach	Tarragon, thyme, oregano, rosemary
Squash	Basil, dill, oregano, savory
Tomatoes	Basil, oregano, dill, garlic, savory, parsley, bay leaf

Book
Two

Muscular Conditioning

CHAPTER FIFTEEN

MUSCULAR CONDITIONING

Those who think they have not time for bodily exercise will sooner or later have to find time for illness.
—Edward Stanley

Now that we understand the nutritional needs for maintaining Whole Health, let's move on to the next component of the Whole Health Equation: muscular conditioning.

In order to exercise our bodies most efficiently, it's important to have an understanding of the part of the body we want to condition: the muscles.

WHAT MAKES A MUSCLE?

Over 430 voluntary muscles (muscles controlled by will) can be identified in the body. The tissue of these muscles is made up of thousands of elongated, cylindrical cells called muscle fibers. These fibers are encased by a sheath of connective tissue called the sarcolemma. If you removed one of these fibers for close examination, you would find that it is composed of many long, parallel strands called myofibrils. The myofibrils are responsible for the actual lengthening and contracting of the muscles. Once our body has totally matured, we are left with a certain number of muscle fibers determined by our genetic heritage.

In performing progressive resistance exercises, exercises where free weights and machines are used at successively greater levels of resistance, we can increase the strength and size of these fibers, and, in turn, increase the strength and size of the

The treadmill stress test is an effective way to measure your overall level of cardiovascular fitness, as well as determine if you have a condition that needs special attention. You may even want to have your body fat percentage measured. Body fat percentages can accurately be determined by the use of either skin fold measurements using calipers or hydrostatic (underwater) weighing. Seeing the change in the results of such tests can be quite motivating.

BLOOD PROFILES

Regardless of your age or level of fitness, I strongly encourage you to have a blood profile done. A blood draw is a simple procedure that can be performed in as little as 10 minutes. Yet the results of this test are invaluable. As I said earlier, some people can look deceptively healthy on the outside while on the inside disease is taking its toll. A blood profile is like a window on the inside of the body that allows us to see what's really going on with our health.

Blood profiles contain values for numerous components. Those with which we are most concerned include your total cholesterol, HDL cholesterol, triglycerides, and glucose. As we saw in the nutrition chapters, your blood cholesterol level is a strong indicator of your risk for coronary heart disease and stroke. The higher your total cholesterol, the higher your risk for such diseases. However, total cholesterol is not the only factor to be concerned with. HDL (high-density lipoprotein) cholesterol is also an important indicator. As we have seen, a higher HDL level has been associated with a lower risk for heart disease.

Triglycerides are fats or lipids stored for energy. Their level indicates how well your body processes fats. Abnormally high triglyceride levels are also a risk factor for heart disease.

Glucose represents the sugar in blood. Adequate blood sugar levels are essential for abundant energy and proper function of all the organs of the body, particularly the brain. Excessively low levels of glucose, or what is known as hypoglycemia, can be a significant problem. Excessively high levels of blood glucose can indicate a risk of diabetes.

AGE FACTORS

Among people age 65 and older, more than two of every five
report essentially sedentary lifestyles.
– American Heart Association

There is no "right" age to begin an exercise program. I always say the sooner the better. While the response to exercise will vary from individual to individual, everyone can enhance his or her level of fitness, regardless of age. It seems that between the ages of 16 and 25, individuals experience the most immediate muscle growth and recuperation when performing progressive resistance exercises and that, after about 45 years of age, increases in strength and muscle mass *may* be more difficult to come by. However, these are averages and are by no means carved in stone! I don't believe there is a cut-off age for exercise either. I have seen men and women in their seventies who exercise regularly, some with physiques that would make persons half their age green with envy!

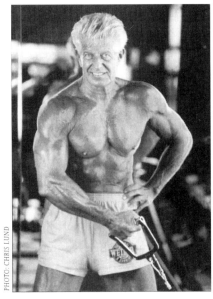

PHOTO: CHRIS LUND

At 75, Bob Delmonteque is living proof of the benefits of lifelong exercise.

PROGRESSIVE RESISTANCE TRAINING		
WEEK 1	Day 1	Day 2	Day 3

WEEK 1	Day 1	Day 2	Day 3
SET A	75 x 8	75 x 10	75 x 11
SET B	75 x 8	75 x 9	75 x 9
SET C	75 x 8	75 x 8	75 x 9

WEEK 2	Day 1	Day 2	Day 3
SET A	75 x 12	75 x 12	75 x 12
SET B	75 x 11	75 x 12	75 x 12
SET C	75 x 10	75 x 11	75 x 12

WEEK 3	Day 1	Day 2	Day 3
SET A	80 x 9	80 x 10	80 x 11
SET B	80 x 9	80 x 9	80 x 11
SET C	80 x 8	80 x 8	80 x 9

WEEK 4	Day 1	Day 2	Day 3
SET A	80 x 11	80 x 12	85 x 10
SET B	80 x 11	80 x 12	85 x 8
SET C	80 x 10	80 x 12	85 x 8

3 sets of 8-12 repetitions with 75-85 lb. weights.

WOMEN'S CONCERNS

While the advice in this book is, for the most part, equally directed toward both men and women, there are a number of concerns that pertain exclusively to women, which I present below.

WOMEN, STRENGTH, AND MUSCLE

While the physiological responses to exercise of men and women are comparable, the rate and degree to which those responses occur differ because of certain gender-oriented predispositions.

For instance, it is very likely that if we were to expose a man and a woman to the exact same training program, the man would develop muscle at a faster rate and to a greater degree than the woman. The reason for this is that men have significantly higher levels of the hormone *testosterone*, which is responsible for the manufacture of the contractile proteins of muscle. While a woman might put equal time and intensity into her training, ultimately, she will see less dramatic growth in her musculature. This is not to say that women cannot develop muscles and strength, because they certainly can. (One look at the biceps my mother acquired in four months is a confirmation of that!) Rather, it's important that women understand their unique physiological makeup so they can more effectively plan for and appreciate their exercise experience.

WOMEN, BODY FAT LEVELS, AND AMENORRHEA

Another important concern is body fat levels or percentages. Some women are unaware of the fact that, because of their reproductive needs, they *naturally* carry more fat or adipose tissue than men. A woman's body makes sure it has the stored energy to meet the demands of pregnancy, should there be a scarcity of food. Typically, an average woman will carry 6 percent more fat than an average man. This difference is consistent even in top-form male and female athletes. Women carry higher levels of fat for good reason, and they should not expect to reach

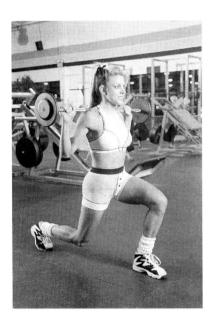

excessively low levels (8-12 percent) without incurring some side effects. One such side effect is amenorrhea, the cessation of the menstrual cycle.

Although temporary amenorrhea can be caused by a variety of factors, it is not an uncommon consequence in women whose body fat levels have dropped to abnormally low levels. This is sometimes referred to as exercise-associated amenorrhea or EAA. There are no reports that show this to be a dangerous condition as long as it is temporary, and in most cases, the problem can be corrected simply by increasing body weight and/or reducing training intensity levels. Long-term amenorrhea may be indicative of a more serious problem and may increase a woman's risk of developing osteoporosis. In such cases, a woman should consult her healthcare provider. On the more positive side, women who participate in a regular exercise program report that they have shorter menstrual cycles and experience fewer cramps and less of the discomfort associated with menstruation.

EXERCISE AND PREGNANCY

Understandably, a pregnant mother wants to take every precaution. In most cases, with certain limitations, she can continue to exercise. In fact, a strong back and conditioned cardiovascular system are quite beneficial to pregnancy, labor, and the birth process. Research shows that women who exercise regularly have shorter and easier labor due to their increased level of endurance.[105] Given that a woman has undergone a thorough prenatal exam, the American College of Obstetricians and Gynecologists recommends that exercise sessions be limited to 15 minutes and that the woman's heart rate not exceed 140 beats per minute. Techniques for measuring heart rate will be discussed in the aerobics section.

As a pregnancy progresses, natural changes will eventually prevent the mother from participating fully in an exercise program. Primarily, this is due to a change in the center of gravity caused by the growing fetus. Certain sports, because of jarring impact or the risk of falling, should be avoided, including running or jogging, horseback riding, water-skiing, and scuba diving. Sit-ups are also to be avoided. Ideal activities include swimming, brisk walking, and stretching. Some health clubs are now offering aerobic classes specifically designed for pregnant women.

THE FEAR OF "BIGNESS"

A final concern regards the fear of "bigness." Although I have had a number of male clients address this issue, it is most often a woman who says, "I want to exercise with weights, but I don't want to get big." I usually respond to this statement by pointing out that nobody "gets big" overnight. The fear of getting too big is really unwarranted. The kind of size associated with power lifters or professional bodybuilders comes from many years of extremely hard training with excessively heavy weights. Always remember, there is a direct relationship between the size of a muscle and the degree of resistance it must contract against. In other words, heavy weights are required to elicit the kind of muscle growth a power lifter or competitive bodybuilder desires. Light to moderate weights and the higher repetitions they allow for, are more effective for toning and strengthening and less effective for developing significant size. Further, as I mentioned in the Introduction, muscle hypertrophy (growth) occurs at a gradual rate (much slower than some would like). For this reason, it is possible for each of us to continually monitor our bodies and the effects exercise is having on them. If we are not happy with the direction in which we are moving, we can redirect our efforts toward the results we desire.

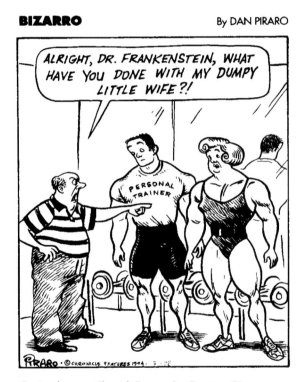

Reprinted courtesy Chronicle Features, San Francisco, CA.

CHAPTER SEVENTEEN

THE STRETCHING PROGRAM

Either you reach a higher point today, or you exercise your strength in order to be able to climb higher tomorrow.
– Friedrich Wilhelm Nietzche

Before looking at the pre-conditioning program in the next chapter, I want to communicate the importance of stretching and provide you with a complete stretching program. The combination of the pre-conditioning program and the stretching exercises will help to increase your flexibility, strength, and coordination, priming you for the exercise routines in the beginning and intermediate chapters.

STRETCHING

Stretching is not complex or difficult; it merely needs to be practiced regularly. In addition to reducing the risk of injury, a regular stretching program will relieve stress and tension, increase body awareness, and most important, increase circulation. The wonderful thing about stretching is that it requires no equipment and can be done just about anyplace, at any time. There are countless stretches that one can do, some as basic as those taught in high school physical education classes, others more elaborate. The stretches I have included here are the ones I believe are most effective for overall conditioning.

When performing a stretch, ease into the movement rather than bounce or jerk your way through. Too often I see individuals (even professional athletes!) perform ballistic stretches in which they bounce or lurch. These same people often lack flexibility. The reason is that ballistic movements put one head-to-head with a physiological response known as the stretch reflex. This response, a sudden contraction of the muscle being stretched, is a protective reaction that serves to prevent potential tissue damage. The fibers responsible for this response are called the muscle spindles. During a static stretch, where the movement is progressive and controlled, the spindle accompanies the muscle fibers in their elongation. Yet, as soon as it detects movement that could be dangerous, it locks. To avoid this lock-up response, your stretch movements should always be controlled and fluid. At the first sign of tension or resistance, you should stop. Hold the position (usually for 15-30 seconds) until the pull has subsided, and then continue to move further into the stretch until the pull is felt again. While stretching, you may become tense and either hold your breath or breathe shallowly. This will counteract your efforts. Be sure to make a conscious effort to breathe deeply, as this will facilitate your stretching. The distance you move in a stretch could be two inches or two millimeters. What's important is that you focus on the feeling, not how far you move. Flexibility comes gradually, and the process should never be painful, so don't become frustrated if you can't drop into the splits after a week!

Stretching should be performed before every exercise session, but can be helpful at other times, as well. When stretching before exercise, be sure to warm up your muscles first by performing some light activity such as walking or pedaling a stationary bicycle with no resistance. You can stretch after your exercise session, as a way of "warming down" and to reduce the likelihood of soreness from training. Try to get in the habit of stretching whenever you think about it, while talking on the phone, watching television, or even while you're in the bathtub.

THE STRETCHES

Hamstring stretch

Sit on the floor and pull either your left or right leg inward so that the sole of your foot rests next to the inside of the thigh of the extended leg (Fig. 1). Slowly, and from the hip, begin to bend forward in the direction of the foot of the extended leg. As soon as you feel resistance, stop and hold that position for 15-30 seconds. Once the resistance has subsided, continue forward again until the pulling feeling returns. Hold this position again for about 15 seconds. Then, stretch the hamstrings of the other leg in the same manner.

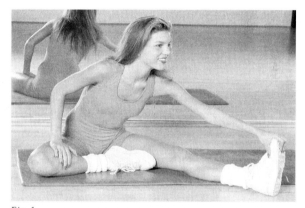

Fig. 1

Lower back and hip stretch

This is one of my favorite stretches for the lower back. Most people find an immediate release of lower back tension when performing this stretch.

While lying on your back, bend one knee into a 90-degree angle. Using the hand of your opposite side and placing the palm on the outside of the knee, pull the leg over toward the floor (Fig. 2). Turn your head to the opposite direction of your bent knee. Relax and hold this position for 15-30 seconds. Switch legs and repeat. Don't be concerned if you are unable to touch the floor with your knee.

There is no need to force your knee down, either. With time you will gain an increased range of motion.

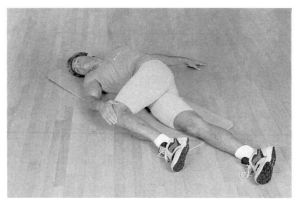

Fig.2

Groin stretch

Sitting with the soles of your feet facing each other, and your knees facing out to the sides, hold your feet together, and move forward from the hips. Pause when you encounter resistance and hold 15-30 seconds (Fig. 3). Be sure not to round your back in this movement.

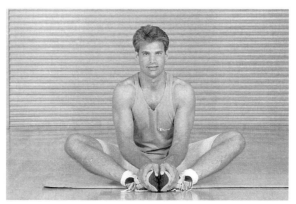

Fig.3

Hip-flexor stretch

This stretch will primarily affect the iliopsoas muscles (also known as the hip flexors) located at the front of the hip and may also be felt in the hamstring and groin areas.

While keeping your right foot flat on the floor and using your hands to support you, bend your right knee and extend your left leg behind you. Your knee should be directly above your right ankle. Rest your left knee on the floor. Then allow your hip to move toward the floor for 15-30 seconds (Fig. 4). Repeat this movement with your left foot forward. Be sure that the knee of the forward leg is always aligned over the ankle.

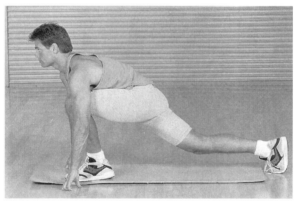

Fig.4

Cobra stretch

Lie on your stomach with your hands shoulders-width apart. Gently, push your torso up, exhaling as you go. Hold the stretch for about 15 seconds. Be sure to keep your hips against the floor at all times (Fig. 5).

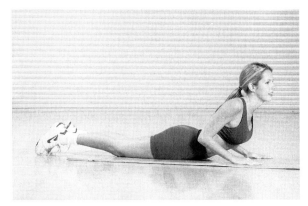

Fig. 5

Thigh stretch

This movement will stretch the powerful quadricep muscles of the leg. Stand near a wall for stability. Lift either leg behind you, grasp your ankle, and gently pull your leg up behind you. Gradually, bring your heel close to your buttocks and hold this position for 15-30 seconds. To enhance the stretch effect, tilt your pelvis forward by contracting your abdominal muscles, then extend the pelvis by contracting your buttocks (Fig. 6). Repeat with your other leg.

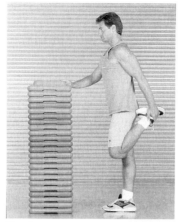

Fig.6

Calf stretch

Stand facing a wall or other sturdy structure at arm's length. While keeping one knee straight, place the foot of the other leg in front of you, toes toward the wall (Fig. 7). The rear leg should be kept straight with the heel on the floor. With your forearms against the wall and elbows bent, slowly move forward from the hip. When you feel a pull in the calf of your straight leg, hold the position for 15-30 seconds. Do this stretch on both sides.

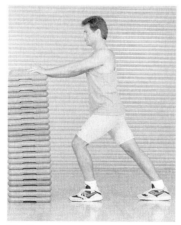

Fig.7

Low-back stretch

Lie flat on your back. With your fingers interlaced under your knee, pull your thigh in toward your chest to increase the stretch. Hold this position for about 15-30 seconds (Fig. 8). Switch legs and repeat the movement. This stretch is very relaxing for the lower back and creates an "opening" action in the hips. This movement can also be performed with both legs simultaneously.

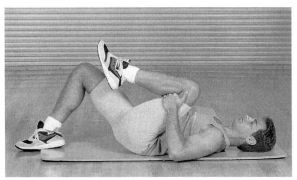

Fig.8

Cat stretch

Instinctively, cats perform a stretch similar to this several times a day. Kneel on the floor making sure to keep your knees under your hips and your hands under your shoulders. Exhale as you round your back, holding the position for 15-30 seconds. This stretch (Fig. 9) can be used interchangeably with the cow stretch.

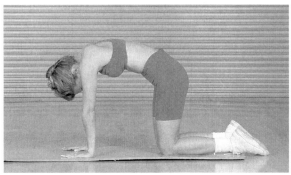

Fig.9

Cow stretch

Kneel on the floor positioning your knees and hands the same as in the cat stretch. Exhale as you arch your back gently (Fig. 10).

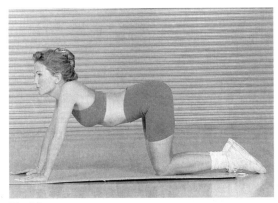

Fig. 10

Tricep stretch

As if you were scratching your shoulder, put your right or left arm behind your back. Then, place your opposite hand on top of your elbow. Slowly push the elbow down, until you feel a stretch in the tricep. Hold this stretch for about 15-30 seconds, then repeat with the other arm. A variation of this stretch involves using either a broomstick or a towel (Fig. 11).

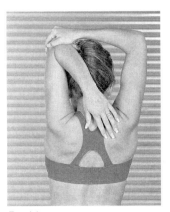
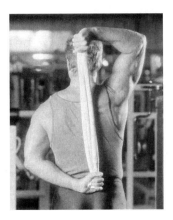

Fig. 11

Back stretch

This is a great movement for stretching out the latissimus muscles of the back. Kneel on the floor with your forehead resting on your left forearm (Fig. 12). Extend your right arm straight forward. While pressing lightly with your extended palm, pull yourself back slowly. Hold for 15-30 seconds. Perform this stretch on both sides.

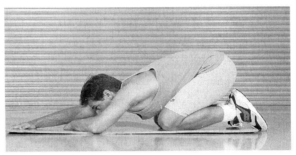

Fig.12

Chest-shoulder stretch

While standing or sitting, grasp a towel or broomstick with an overhand grip, a medium to wide width (Fig. 13). Raise your arms above your body. Then, slowly lower the towel or stick behind your back. To alter the degree of stretch felt in the chest, vary the width of your grip. Hold for about 15-30 seconds. A similar stretch can be performed by placing your forearms upright on either side of a doorway and then gently moving forward through the doorway.

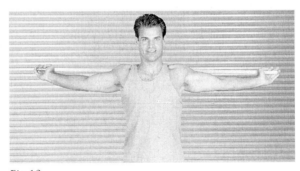

Fig.13

Sit up with your back erect and your legs extended in front of you. Bend your right leg, and place your right foot on the outside of your left knee. Then place your left elbow against the outside of your right knee. Use your other hand to support you as you twist to the rear, exhaling as you go. Repeat on the other side (Fig. 14).

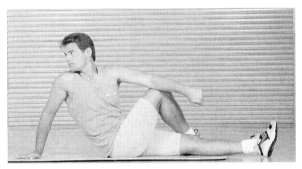

Fig. 14

Full body stretch

This is a wonderful all-body stretch. Lie on your back with your arms extended beyond your head and legs fully extended. Reach with both your hands and feet in opposite directions, simultaneously (Fig. 15). Hold this reach for about 15 seconds and relax. Repeat two to three times.

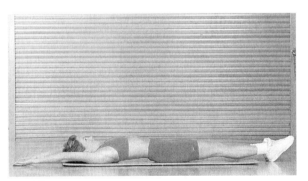

Fig. 15

Remember, stretching is not a competitive sport and you needn't try to outperform someone else. Each of us has a different degree of flexibility, and the rate at which our flexibility increases varies greatly. Within a short period of time, you'll see a dramatic improvement in yours! Some days you may be more flexible than others. If you find that you are particularly tight one day, don't worry. Simply spend a bit more time on the stretches, continue to be consistent, and you will progress.

If you have the time, perform these stretches after your workout, as well as before, and at any other time you can. I find that stretching before bed is an excellent way to "wind down" and accelerate my ability to enter into deep sleep.

CHAPTER EIGHTEEN

THE PRE-CONDITIONING PROGRAM

The human body is the best picture of the human soul.
– Ludwig Wittgenstein

If you were to take a look at some of the skyscrapers in the downtown area of your city, you'd see some spectacular structures, each possessing an elaborate facade of marble and other materials that make it seem invulnerable. However, each of these buildings has deep within itself a "skeleton" system of I-beams, rebar, and concrete that creates the infrastructure of the building. Without a well-built infrastructure for support, somewhere down the road, whether due to age or natural catastrophe, a building may encounter structural problems. The same goes for an exercise program. The pre-conditioning program is about laying a solid foundation for your exercise program.

The beginning stages are the most important part of conditioning the body. If you don't start out properly, working on the fundamentals of a strong foundation, you're making a compromise. This is one of the greatest pitfalls of those just beginning an exercise program. They often try to take on intermediate or even advanced level exercise with little or no prior experience. I know a man who ran in a marathon (that's over 26 miles) because he thought it would "get him in shape." He had almost no running experience at all prior to the race. He volunteered that after the race he "walked funny" for a week. He was fortunate; things could have been far worse. I regularly see newcomers to exercise "attack" enormous amounts of weight on exercise machines, and try to break records on stationary cycles.

PULL-UPS

Pull-ups are an excellent exercise for overall back development. If you had to choose only one exercise to do for your back, this would be it! Pull-ups also place secondary emphasis on the biceps.

For this exercise you will need access to a pull-up bar. I know I said you wouldn't need to purchase any equipment, so let's look at your options. Many communities have "par courses" or jogging tracks on roadsides or through parks that have exercise stations along their path. Often included among these stations is a pull-up bar, usually consisting of wood posts with a bar in between. If you are inclined to buy a bar, there are inexpensive pull-up bars that are portable and fit into any doorway. They cost around $15.

Begin with an overhand grip about shoulders-width apart. Starting with arms fully extended, body hanging, pull yourself up until your chin is above the bar (Fig. 16). Slowly, lower yourself back to the hanging position, allowing for a full stretch in the "lat" muscles.

Your goal should be to work toward performing 30 pull-ups, yet doing even two your first workout may be tough. Don't be discouraged. I have worked with many beginners who have been unable to perform a single pull-up on their first attempt. Yet, in a few weeks they could perform sets with considerable ease.

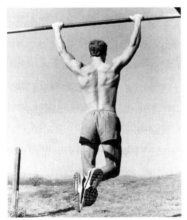
Fig.16 Start

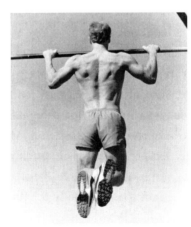
Fig.16 Finish

PUSH-UPS

This is a great exercise for the entire upper body. When performed properly, it benefits not only the chest muscles, but also the shoulders, triceps, and even the abdominals.

Once while working on a film production, two burly stagehands asked me to join them in a little fun. They wanted to have a push-up contest. Judging from the shape these guys appeared to be in, I assumed they'd be able to breeze through 50 or 60 push-ups easily. Nevertheless, I was game. While in the midst of our little contest, I glanced over and watched the other two men. One had his buttocks sticking up in the air so high he looked more like a right angle touching his forehead to the floor. The other had gone through a radical change. Having started on the ends of his toes, he was now on his knees doing "stomach-ups." Although this was all in good fun, I called time and confronted these "he-men" about their form. They weren't even doing push-ups, I explained. At first they thought I was being a poor sport until I showed them the correct form. Once they tried it, it was a totally different deal. No longer did they want to compete; instead they were intrigued with the difference in the feeling. Now they were seeing that correct form really works the muscles and demands a lot more. I left for a moment, and returned to find the two of them calling each other on form. "Pull that stomach in," and "straighten your back," they were saying. It was a funny sight, but I knew that now, having done some real push-ups, they would never go back to their "cheating ways."

The moral is, of course, that for the full benefit of this exercise, as well as any other, it is imperative that you pay special attention to form. Don't get into the trap of valuing quantity over quality. Ten well-executed push-ups will do far more for your body and the foundation of your exercise program than 50 push-ups that are done improperly. With that in mind, let's begin.

With your hands shoulders-width apart, fingers facing forward, feet about 6 inches apart, lower yourself until your chest touches the floor. Your body should remain rigid, head in alignment with spine, with only your arms bending. Once your chest (not your stomach), has touched the floor, press yourself back up to the point just before your elbows lock (Fig. 17). A wider placement of your hands will direct more stress to the chest, whereas a narrower placement stresses the shoulders and triceps more.

In the beginning, you may be able to do only five or less; if you're in shape, more. With time you'll adapt. Your goal should be 50. Perhaps you'll be able to perform two sets of 25 or five sets of 10. Whatever works for you is fine. After you have gained some strength, for an extra challenge, perform push-ups with your feet elevated on a chair or bed end.

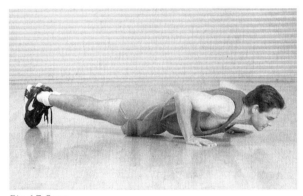

Fig.17 Start

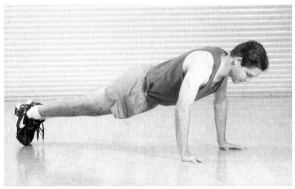

Fig.17 Finish

DIPS

When they are performed in strict fashion, dips primarily develop and strengthen the tricep muscles of the arm, the shoulders, and the lower portion of the chest. You may use a couple of chairs or two exercise benches.

Squat down and place your hands behind you on the seat of one chair or bench edge. Then, extend your legs, resting your heels on the opposite chair. Slowly bend your arms and lower yourself toward the floor. Focusing on the triceps, extend your arms, raising yourself to a point just before your elbows lock. Always stop before locking your elbows and never descend lower than where your upper arms

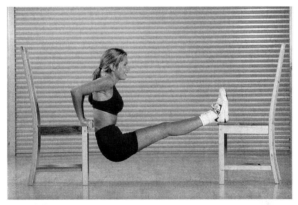

Fig. 18 Start

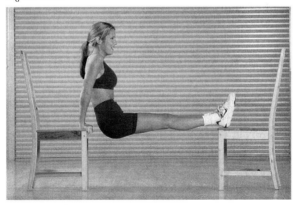

Fig. 18 Finish

are parallel to the floor (Fig. 18). Your goal should be to perform 30. Again, you can do three sets of 10 or any other combination that works for you.

SQUATS

Squats are great for strengthening the powerful quadricep muscles of the thigh. Secondary emphasis is placed on the hamstrings and buttocks. With your feet facing forward and about 12 inches apart, slowly descend into the squat position. Go no further than the point where your thighs are parallel to the floor. Then, raise yourself back to the starting point (Fig. 19).

It's important that you keep your torso as straight and upright as possible throughout the exercise. I suggest you either keep your hands on your hips or extend them straight out in front of you. Some people find it more comfortable to elevate their heels on a 2-inch block of wood. An encyclopedia or other large book

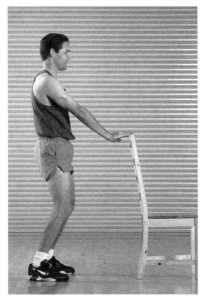 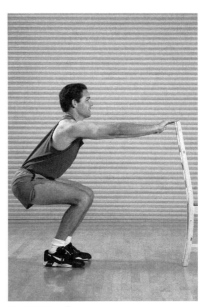

Fig. 19 Start   Fig. 19 Finish

will suffice for this purpose. Your goal should be to perform 75 reps. Three sets of 25 would be a good approach.

HEEL RAISES

Like squats, heel raises can be effectively performed using a large book or other elevated platform to stand on. Begin with the balls of your feet placed on the edge of either the step or sturdy book, and about 5 inches apart. Lifting your heels, raise up on the balls of your feet until the calf muscles are fully contracted. Then lower

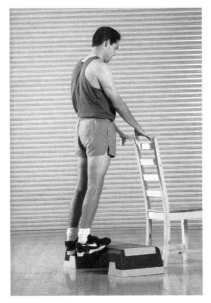
Fig.20 Start

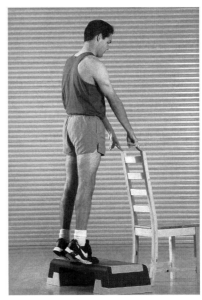
Fig.20 Finish

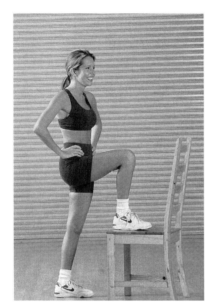 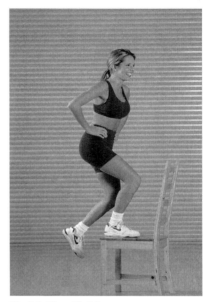

Fig.22 Start  Fig.22 Near Finish

AEROBIC CONDITIONING

The health of the people is really the foundation upon which all their happiness and all their powers as a state depend.
— Benjamin Disraeli

So far, we have examined stretching, calisthenics, and progressive resistance forms of exercise. Now we will look at the other essential component of physical exercise, aerobics.

Aerobic conditioning is generally achieved by performing at moderate intensity exercises that employ larger muscle groups in a rhythmic and continuous fashion for an extended duration (20-60 minutes). Running, cycling, swimming, and cross-country skiing are examples of aerobic exercise. Conversely, high-intensity exercises such as sprinting and using free weights and variable resistance machines are considered *anaerobic* because often oxygen demand exceeds oxygen intake.

The primary goal of regular aerobic exercise is to achieve greater cardiopulmonary or cardiovascular fitness. This means an increased efficiency in the function of the heart (cardio), the lungs (pulmonary), and the blood vessels (vascular). In addition, there are numerous other benefits gained from regular aerobic exercise.

BENEFITS OF AEROBIC EXERCISE

STRENGTHENS THE HEART

The primary benefit of aerobic exercise is its ability to strengthen the cardiovascular system (heart and blood vessels). The heart is a muscle, too. Its job

Center in Washington, D.C., found that even those with severe hypertension could reduce their medication doses by up to 40 percent after only 16 weeks of regular aerobic exercise.

HELPS PREVENT BREAST CANCER

Several epidemiological studies have suggested that physical activity may reduce the risk of breast cancer. The most recent was reported in the *Journal of the National Cancer Institute*.

At the University of Southern California, Dr. Leslie Bernstein and colleagues found that women who participate in four or more hours of physical activity a week (running, swimming, aerobics, weight training) during their reproductive years can reduce their risk for breast cancer by 60 percent, relative to inactive women. It is believed that breast cancer risk increases with exposure to ovarian hormones (estradiol and progesterone). The protection may come from the fact that exercise alters menstrual cycle patterns and the synthesis of these hormones, thereby reducing the degree to which sensitive tissues are exposed to them.

HELPS PREVENT OSTEOPOROSIS

As we have seen, osteoporosis is a condition in which the bones become porous and frail, leading to increased risk of fractures. Again, we have too long accepted this condition as an inevitable part of the aging process. In truth, there is much we can do to retard, if not prevent, this condition.

As I have already mentioned, bone will respond much like muscle, and atrophy with disuse. However, when subjected to weight-bearing exercises, bone size and density tend to increase. Sedentary living reduces the stress on bones, and, much like muscle that is unchallenged, it begins to atrophy, de-mineralize, and become weaker. The National Institutes of Health now recommends a program of weight-bearing exercise as an important means of preventing osteoporosis.

Remember, although sedentary living is one contributing factor in osteoporosis, as we learned in Chapter Five, a high-animal protein and phosphorus diet plays a significant role – much greater than has been considered until now.

HELPS PREVENT DIABETES

Recent findings from the Honolulu Heart Program confirm that those who exercise regularly enjoy a 50 percent reduction in the risk of developing non-insulin-dependent diabetes. Furthermore, in cases where diabetes has already been diagnosed, regular aerobic exercise in conjunction with a low-fat diet has shown dramatic results. In one study, 71 percent of subjects taking an oral hypoglycemic prescription and 39 percent of those taking insulin were able to discontinue their medication after only three weeks of this lifestyle modification program.[108] One of the reasons for such improvement is that exercise can increase the number of

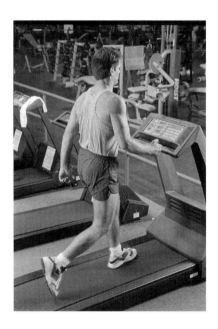

AGE	AGE PREDICTED HEART RATE GUIDE				
	MHR	50%	60%	70%	85%
16	204	102	122	143	173
18	202	101	121	141	172
20	200	100	120	140	170
22	198	99	119	139	168
24	196	98	118	137	166
26	194	97	116	136	165
28	192	96	115	134	163
30	190	95	114	133	161
32	188	94	113	132	160
34	186	93	112	130	158
36	184	92	110	129	156
38	182	91	109	127	155
40	180	90	108	126	153
42	178	89	107	125	151
44	176	88	106	123	150
46	174	87	104	122	148
48	172	86	103	120	146
50	170	85	102	119	145
52	168	84	101	118	143
54	166	83	100	116	141
56	164	82	98	115	139
58	162	81	97	113	138
60	160	80	96	112	136
62	158	79	95	111	134
64	156	78	94	109	133
66	154	77	92	108	131
68	152	76	91	106	129
70	150	75	90	105	128

conditioned, our anaerobic threshold becomes greater, allowing us to exercise at higher intensities and still remain "aerobic" in effect. While training heart rate is important, a reliable method for checking aerobic intensity is called the "talk test." At any time, you should be able to carry on a conversation with another person without feeling winded.

PROPER WARM-UPS

Whatever your target heart rate, you don't want to reach it immediately. It is *imperative* that you warm up before reaching your target heart rate. Warm-ups are any activity performed at a rate of intensity much lower than when exercising. For example, walking, light jogging in place, and stationary cycling are all effective ways to warm up as long as they are performed for three to five minutes at low intensities. A warm-up period allows the body to acclimate in several ways. First,

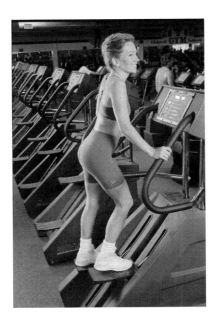

15-WEEK WALKING PROGRAM			
Walk (minutes)	Brisk Walk (minutes)	Walk (minutes)	Total (minutes)
WEEK 1	5	1	5	11
WEEK 2	5	2	5	12
WEEK 3	5	5	5	15
WEEK 4	5	8	5	18
WEEK 5	5	10	5	20
WEEK 6	5	12	5	22
WEEK 7	5	15	5	25
WEEK 8	5	17	5	27
WEEK 9	5	20	5	30
WEEK 10	5	22	5	32
WEEK 11	5	25	5	35
WEEK 12	5	27	5	37
WEEK 13	5	30	5	40
WEEK 14	5	32	5	42
WEEK 15	5	35	5	45

Program should be followed three non-consecutive days.

RUNNING

Running is also an excellent form of aerobic conditioning that helps develop, strengthen, and condition the muscles you are exercising in the gym. A regular running program offers all the same health benefits of the walking program. Today, it is estimated that 30 million Americans include running in their regular exercise program. Caution: If you have any type of orthopedic condition (bone or joint problem), running is probably not your best choice for aerobic exercise.

If you choose to begin running and have no previous experience, I suggest a gradual "break-in" period before you attempt to win any marathons. The best way to start is simply by following the above walking program. As you become more conditioned, instead of brisk walking you can increase your pace to a jogging and then running pace. Jogging is not running. Think of it as a stage between a brisk walking and running pace. Initially, work from a jog/run/jog period to a full running period between your five-minute warm-up and five-minute cool-down periods. I have included a sample running program (see page 276) you may wish to use as a model in fashioning your own running program.

How to Run

Proper running form not only helps prevent injury and premature exhaustion, but will also make your run more enjoyable. First, make sure to keep your shoulders relaxed at all times. There can be a tendency to lift the shoulders and hold them in tensely. When the shoulders are lifted, the arms usually end up pinned to the sides of the body. If the arms are relaxed and free, you can move them forward in a pumping motion. This movement will increase momentum and propel you forward with greater ease. Your hands should be loose (not in a fist) and move directly in

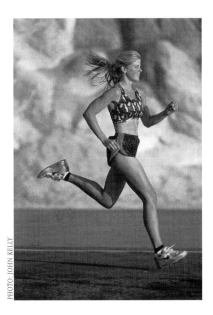

PHOTO: JOHN KELLY

15–WEEK RUNNING PROGRAM		
Walk	Jog/Run/Jog	Walk
WEEK 1 — 5 mins	1 mins	5 mins
WEEK 2 — 5 mins	3 mins	5 mins
WEEK 3 — 5 mins	5 mins	5 mins
WEEK 4 — 5 mins	7 mins	5 mins
WEEK 5 — 5 mins	10 mins	5 mins
WEEK 6 — 5 mins	12 mins	5 mins
WEEK 7 — 5 mins	15 mins	5 mins
WEEK 8 — 5 mins	17 mins	5 mins
WEEK 9 — 5 mins	20 mins	5 mins
WEEK 10 — 5 mins	22 mins	5 mins
WEEK 11 — 5 mins	25 mins	5 mins
WEEK 12 — 5 mins	27 mins	5 mins
WEEK 13 — 5 mins	30 mins	5 mins
WEEK 14 — 5 mins	32 mins	5 mins
WEEK 15 — 5 mins	35 mins	5 mins

Program should be followed three non-consecutive days.

CHAPTER TWENTY

THE BEGINNING PROGRAM

Whatever you can do, or dream you can, begin it.
Boldness has genius, power and magic to it.
– Goethe

By now you have followed the novice program for at least three or four weeks, and you're ready to move on to the beginning level exercises. I'm certain you have noticed some changes taking place in your physique already, particularly if you've been following the guidelines of the Revised American Diet. Your body may be showing a new shape, you're probably stronger, and have increased your level of stamina. I trust you are also enjoying the increased flexibility afforded by your regular stretching (you are stretching, aren't you?). You should feel great about the progress you have made; you're on your way to a life of strength, energy, and overall wellness! Your body should be sufficiently conditioned at this point to move on to the beginning level programs using free weights and machines.

With the exception of a few exercises, the beginning program outlined at the end of this chapter incorporates many of the same movements you have been performing in the novice program, yet now you will perform these exercises with weights for added resistance.

There are two types of exercises in progressive resistance training: basic and isolation. Basic exercises, such as the ones in the beginning routine, are those exercises that work larger muscle groups such as the latissimus (back) and quadriceps (thighs) in accordance with smaller, synergistic muscles such as the biceps, deltoids (shoulders), and trapezius (upper back). On the other hand, isolation exercises (such as the concentration curl, shrug, and fly), when performed in strict form, provide direct stress to a smaller segment of a muscle group. Because there is little help from synergistic or "assistant" muscles, you will likely find isolation exercises more intense. Although you will progressively add new isolation exercises to your repertoire, the basic exercises will always remain a fundamental part of your exercise routine. Basic and isolation exercises for each muscle group are differentiated in the chart below.

BASIC VS. ISOLATION EXERCISES		
	Basic	Isolation
CHEST	Barbell bench press, Incline barbell press, Dumbbell press, Incline dumbbell press, Dips	Flys, Incline flys, Pec-deck flys
SHOULDERS	Upright rows, Behind-the-neck press	Dumbbell lateral raise, Frontal raise, Bent-over lateral raise
BICEPS	Standing barbell curl, Dumbbell curl, Preacher curl	Concentration curl
TRICEPS	Lying barbell tricep extension, Dips, Close-grip bench press	Cable push downs, Dumbbell kickback
BACK	Barbell row, Dumbbell row, Seated cable row, Pull-downs, Pull-ups	Shrug, Back extension
LEGS	Squat, Leg press, Lunge	Leg extension, Leg curl
FOREARMS	Barbell reverse-grip curl	Barbell wrist curl

CAUTION TO BEGINNERS

I cannot overstate the importance of listening to your own inner wisdom in exercising. Though our bodies have much in common, each of us will have a unique response to diet and exercise.

For example, two people could be riding stationary bicycles next to one another, yet one may be pedaling at a higher RPM or utilizing greater resistance. However, if both individuals are exercising at their appropriate target heart rate, each will benefit from his efforts. I have often had people tell me they feel compelled to increase the resistance level on the stair climber or stationary cycle when someone next to them begins exercising at a higher rate of intensity. This is why I sometimes tell clients to cover all of the indicator lights on training machines. In truth, the only thing that really matters is your heart rate. The same phenomenon also happens when working with free weights and machines. Individuals sometimes attempt to exercise with greater poundages than they can safely handle in the presence of others. If you find yourself tempted to do this, stop and think about the consequences. While you may or may not impress someone else, you are likely to cause yourself injury.

Strengthening and conditioning the body is a progressive process; it takes time, and no two people will respond to exercise in exactly the same way. As with any sport, there are days when your performance may lag and periods when you may feel you're making little progress. Don't be discouraged. Sometimes noticeable changes may seem painfully slow, but they will happen! Continuous dedication to training and diet will pull you through any slump. And, if you stick with it, you'll come out stronger both physically and mentally. Most important, be intelligent in your exercising. You know inside what is right for you. Listen to your body, as it will guide you in the right direction. With time, you will have acquired the level of fitness you desire, and you will have done so safely!

EXERCISE: WHERE TO DO IT

While it is possible to exercise in your own home, a thorough workout requires that you have access to a variety of equipment. It can become quite expensive trying to outfit a home gym, and the rate at which new, more efficient equipment is being produced could make it very costly to keep up with the progress in technology. Furthermore, much of the equipment that is advertised for home use is often of inferior quality and limited in what it can offer. For the money you might spend on one of the all-in-one machines currently being promoted on television and in magazines, you could purchase at least a year's membership at any one of numerous health club facilities. There you will have access to a vast array of the latest advances in equipment, as well as other possible amenities such as a swimming pool, sauna, and whirlpool. Even if you just won your state's lottery jackpot, there are some other factors to consider about home training. If you have already tried exercising at home, you may have realized how difficult it can be to concentrate with dogs barking, phones ringing, and the constant temptation to cut the workout short and head for the fridge. Additionally, it's unlikely that you'll have a spotter (someone to assist you with the weights) when you need assistance.

One of the reasons I prefer gyms and health clubs, for myself and my clients, is because of the positive effect working out in a group setting has on one's state of mind and performance.

Beware, though! Not all of these places provide a conducive training environment. The atmosphere of a gym or health club can have a strong effect on your mood and your performance during your workout. The range and types of equipment the club provides is also a consideration. For all these reasons, it's advisable that you investigate the various facilities available to you. Take a couple of trial workouts at different times of the day. Most gyms will allow you to do so.

Here are a few other things to consider. How crowded is the facility at peak hours (usually 5-8 p.m.)? This is important, particularly if that's when you plan to be there. Also, some gyms have gigantic memberships (more than 1,000 members), which can make it difficult to access equipment (let alone walk freely) during morning and early evening hours. Therefore, inquire about the gym's membership size. Examine the equipment that is available at the facility. Is it clean and well-maintained? Are there machines "out of order" and in need of repair? Are there enough pieces of equipment available so that you won't have to wait for access to them? How about adequate ventilation? Some clubs are more family-oriented while others may be more hard-core, catering to the "no guts, no glory" types. How about a ride on the stationary cycle with heavy metal music screaming in the background? This is another factor to consider, since many clubs are playing rock and roll music. To some, this is motivating; to others, it's a major distraction. Find a place that inspires you – you'll know it — it will feel right!

TRAINING ATTIRE

You will see an amazing array of athletic wear worn in clubs today. It can be seductive, revealing, and in some cases, "space age." At times, the atmosphere can feel more like a fashion show than a health club. My advice is that you wear as little as possible. This is not to suggest that you train naked, but that the less you wear, the more you will be able to see your body and make an honest assessment of your progress. Undoubtedly, you will see individuals (most often men) who train in all sorts of apparel, including oversized T-shirts, army fatigues, hiking boots, lumberjack shirts, or multiple sweatshirts. When your body is hidden underneath a full Kerolyn warm-up suit or any of the above apparel, it becomes easy to neglect what you can't see. It's difficult to watch your exercise form as well. Lots of bulky clothing restricts your range of motion while exercising, and may become snagged or trapped in the exercise machines. Most health clubs now have pro shops where you can find a wide assortment of appropriate exercise clothing.

WHEN TO EXERCISE

There is no universal "right time" to work out. It's really a matter of personal preference. Some people are at their best in the evenings, whereas others are too tired at the end of the day and prefer an early morning workout. If you work a

eat, the types of food yo
performance and mood. You
and this will be a terrific in

A simple spiral note pac
so that you will remember

Undoubtedly you will
activities into their workou
while exercising. Some w
workout. On several occasio
the newspaper between sets
a set? Probably on the stocl
cartoon section.

CHAPTER TWENTY-ONE

THE INTERMEDIATE PROGRAM

Life is not merely living but living in health.
– Martial

By now, if you have applied the Pre-conditioning and Beginning programs successively, your body should be well conditioned and ready to move on to the Intermediate routines. Undoubtedly, you have noticed great changes taking place in your physique. In fact, it is during the Beginner's Program that the most immediate changes occur. Your toned muscles, definition, and increased strength and flexibility are signs of your progress and should indicate that you are on your way to achieving the strong and healthy physique you desire.

Because new exercises are introduced in this chapter, it will no longer be efficient for you to train your entire body in one session. For this reason I introduce an example of a split routine. In this split routine you will be training the body four times a week rather than three; yet each muscle group will be trained only twice a week so as to assure a sufficient recuperative period. Your training days will be Monday/Thursday and Tuesday/Friday. The remaining three days a week will be reserved for rest and recuperation and some sort of aerobic activity.

By following a split routine schedule, you will be able to focus more intensely on the specific muscle groups you train each day. On Mondays and Thursdays you will exercise chest, shoulders, and triceps; on Tuesdays and Fridays you'll be exercising the legs, back, and biceps. The different muscle groups can be separated in a variety of ways, but I believe that this is the most efficient way. On Monday and Thursday you will be performing those exercises that require pushing or

PHOTO: PAULA CRANE

someone who inspires y

when you're not feeling

be there to encourage yo

"Come on, you're strong

motivating.

Finding a dependable

people who seem more i

You may have to take a

dependable and who has

I would like to stress

carrying one around in th

keep some sort of record

- blood pr
- resting a
- importai
- results f(
- fluctuati
- a careful
- notes ab
- your lon

The value of the diai

find the proof of your po

by referring to your dia

and efficient workouts (

this process of reference

not working in your tra

control over unhealthy e

HIGH-INTENSITY EXERCISE TECHNIQUES

A healthy body is the guest chamber of the soul, a sick, its prison.
— Francis Bacon

In this chapter we will explore more advanced methods of exercising that are commonly employed by athletes and non-athletes who wish to bring greater intensity to their workouts. I am not suggesting that these techniques are for everyone. While sufficient levels of training intensity can be adequately achieved by employing the exercise routines and methods presented thus far, some individuals, particularly athletes, choose to push themselves beyond their normal training threshold. In an effort to elicit a more dramatic change in their muscles' strength, size, and endurance, they will often employ advanced training techniques such as those presented in this chapter. Depending on your current level of fitness and your long-term fitness goals, you may wish to explore some of these advanced fitness strategies yourself.

CIRCUIT TRAINING

Originally, circuit training employed only anaerobic exercises as a means of increasing strength; yet because of how the exercises are performed, the exerciser experienced a moderate aerobic effect. In time, circuits were being performed with aerobic exercises as well.

Circuit training involves designating between 10 and 20 "exercise stations" around the gym where you will perform exercises for each muscle group. The intent is to move from station to station as quickly as possible, resting only during the time it takes for you to get to the next station (about 15 seconds). At each station you perform your 8-12 repetitions, and then move on to the next. After you have completed your full circuit you can take a two– or three-minute rest. You can begin by completing the circuit two or three times just to get used to the feeling and to allow your body to adapt. The key to acquiring the aerobic effect, of course, is to maintain a target heart rate (between 60-85 percent of your maximum rate). Progressively work up until you are completing the circuit four or five times a workout, three times a week.

Aerobic circuits are done the same way except that they employ only aerobic exercises, such as the stationary cycle, rower, stair climber, and the like. Aerobic circuits usually have four to eight stations with performance at each station lasting about three minutes.

CIRCUIT TRAINING ROUTINE		
1. SQUAT	5. WRIST CURL	9. CALF RAISE
2. BENCH PRESS	6. LEG CURL	10. DUMBBELL ROW
3. PULL-UP	7. CRUNCH	11. FLY
4. LATERAL RAISE	8. BARBELL CURL	12. TRICEP EXTENSION

This sample routine is designed using free-weight exercises.
Circuit training can be performed with either free-weights or machines.

NEGATIVE REPS

Negative reps are one way of intensifying your routine. This type of rep places more emphasis on the negative or eccentric contraction of the muscle than on the positive or concentric contraction. Usually, at the point of muscle failure, a complete positive or concentric contraction of the muscle is impossible. However, eccentric or negative repetitions can still be performed with some assistance. It is the eccentric contraction that yields greater muscular force output, and consequently, greater increases in strength.

Negative reps can also be included as part of a regular set prior to muscle failure. In performing these, the goal is to make the downward or negative movement take at least twice as long as the upward or positive movement. If you have already reached a point of muscle failure while training it will be necessary for you to have a partner lift the weight for you and then allow you to perform the negative portion of the movement.

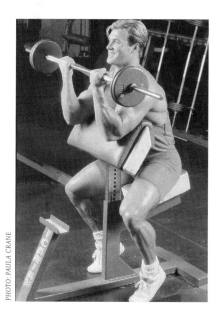

PHOTO: PAULA CRANE

FORCED REPS

Another way of moving beyond the point of temporary muscle failure is to incorporate forced reps into your set. In order to perform forced reps you should have a training partner, or somebody willing to give you some assistance.

During the last reps when muscle failure is likely, your partner can lighten the load on the muscles by pulling up on the barbell or, in the case of dumbbells, by pushing underneath the elbows. With the assistance of just a couple of fingers, your partner can reduce the weight load by a couple of pounds so that you can then complete the rep yourself. It is important that the person helping you not lift the bar for you, but simply reduce the weight slightly, to allow your continuous fluid movement.

STRIPPING

Stripping allows the exerciser to reach temporary muscle failure repeatedly and thereby fatigue a greater number of muscle fibers. This intensification technique is not very popular when exercising with free weights because it requires the assistance of two spotters and, unless you train in a group of three, you may find it difficult to solicit the assistance of two people for this purpose. However, if you can get the assistance, or you are using exercise machines, this is a worthwhile technique.

As an example of the stripping technique, imagine you are doing bench presses and find that you can no longer complete a full repetition with 150 pounds. At this point, each partner or assistant would strip a five-pound plate from the bar, reducing the total poundage to 140 pounds. You may then be able to squeeze out two to three more reps.

BURNS

Burns work particularly well in combination with isolation movements like the concentration curl or leg extensions, but can be applied to almost all movements. Burns are really partial reps performed either at the top or bottom portion of a rep. When you can't complete a full rep alone, you can perform partial reps, moving the weight as far as possible and then returning it to the starting position. The idea is to do as many burns as possible in a quick and successive manner. This really fatigues the muscle and causes a burning sensation for which the movement is named.

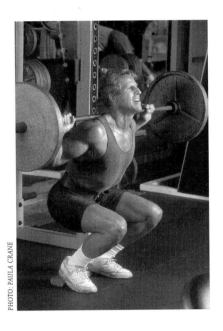

PHOTO: PAULA CRANE

CONCENTRATED REPS

Concentrated reps or what has been called "10-second training," is another intensification technique. Although concentration on your exercise performance is always important, this technique employs a slow and deliberate movement. Each repetition should take about 10 seconds to perform, hence the name. By doing your repetitions in this manner, you will eliminate any of the momentum that might otherwise assist in the lift, and thereby increase the workload to the muscle significantly. Training in this manner usually brings temporary muscle failure very quickly. Like the other intensification techniques, this is very taxing and is best used periodically.

SUPERSETS

A superset is the process of combining two different exercises. There are two superset variations that can be performed: same muscle and opposing muscle. An example of a same muscle superset would be standing barbell curls and preacher curls for the biceps. An example of an opposing muscle superset would be leg extensions in tandem with leg curls.

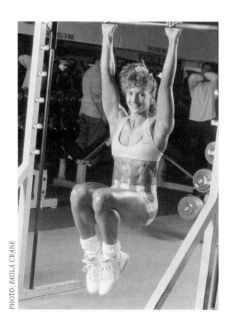

PHOTO: PAULA CRANE

Several things happen when you do supersets. First, you save time. By supersetting two or even three muscle groups that might normally be trained in single sets with rest periods in between, you save a significant amount of rest time. Each muscle group gets rest while you train the other one (the biceps rest while you train the triceps). Another interesting characteristic of supersetting is the feeling of having two or more muscle groups fatigued at the same time (the three heads of the deltoid muscles or the quadriceps and the hamstrings of the legs, for example).

SAMPLE SUPERSET	
1. BARBELL CURL	1 X 8-12 (NO REST)
2. LYING TRICEP EXTENSION	1 X 8-12
	REST
1. BARBELL CURL	1 X 8-12 (NO REST)
2. LYING TRICEP EXTENSION	1 X 8-12
	REST

This sequence is continued until the required number of sets has been performed.

A simple superset of the biceps and triceps would work as follows. Begin with a set of the prescribed number of reps of either standing bar curls or lying tricep extensions. When that first set is completed, move directly to the alternate exercise with no rest in between. After one set for each muscle group has been performed (one for the biceps and one for the triceps), one superset has been completed. At this time a short rest can be taken (60 seconds). Then continue on with another superset until the prescribed number of sets is completed.

TRISETS

Trisets move you to the next level of intensity from supersets. Trisets and supersets are both actually very much the same, in that you are performing more than one exercise for a muscle group with no rest in between. In a triset, however, you perform three exercises before taking a rest. A great muscle group to train with trisets is the deltoids, because the muscle has three different "heads" that can be directly exercised.

SAMPLE TRISET	
1. DUMBBELL FRONTAL RAISE	1 X 8-12 (NO REST)
2. DUMBBELL LATERAL RAISE	1 X 8-12 (NO REST)
3. BENT-OVER LATERAL RAISE	1 X 8-12
REST	
REPEAT	

PYRAMID SETS

Pyramid sets are a very popular technique for intensifying training and rapidly building strength. Pyramid training involves doing several sets of an exercise and consistently increasing the poundages between each set. So far, you have been performing your exercises with a "fixed resistance" or predetermined poundage that you use for all sets. In pyramiding, you increase the weight or resistance level with each successive set while systematically decreasing the number of repetitions. Pyramid sets are usually employed by those who wish not only greater muscle hypertrophy, but also significant increases in strength. The advantage of doing sets in this manner is that by the time you reach the heavier poundages, your muscles will

PYRAMID SETS	
SET 1	1 X 12
SET 2	1 X 10
SET 3	1 X 8
SET 4	1 X 6
SET 5	1 X 4

be well adapted, and the risk of injury is minimized. The pyramid formula usually involves performing five sets, each with a comfortable rest period (1-1$\frac{1}{2}$ minutes) in between. For example, your first set may involve 12 repetitions with a relatively light weight. In the second set, the weight is increased, usually by 10-20 pounds, and the repetitions are decreased by two to accommodate the increased resistance. This process continues until your fifth set, where you will perform four repetitions utilizing maximum poundages.

STICKING POINTS

Unfortunately, everybody seems to reach a plateau or a temporary period when they feel they are not making progress in their exercise program or moving in the direction they wish. Plateaus or "sticking points" arise for a number of reasons, yet there are remedies to push you through these plateaus and continue your progress. During these periods of little or no apparent progress you may find yourself lacking training energy and enthusiasm for your workouts.

Sometimes, sticking points are simply the result of boredom with a routine. In this case, you should simply change your routine; sometimes just substituting a few exercises will suffice. In other cases, progress slows when the body is just too fatigued. If the muscles are overtrained and there has been insufficient time for recuperation, progress will surely slow, if not cease entirely. Another consideration is the neuromuscular system. Muscles that are trained in the same fashion make adaptations that are sometimes difficult to push beyond unless technique is changed. Following are some suggestions for breaking through a sticking point:

Change Routines

Changing routines seems to be the most effective remedy for sticking points. It is easy for the muscles and the mind to become accustomed to a particular routine, which makes it important to keep your training diversified. Boredom can doom your training. So, if you normally exercise in the morning, try exercising at night. Train your abdominal muscles first instead of last, or try incline bench before flat bench presses. If you have been performing "straight sets" for some time, you may wish to employ pyramid or supersets for a while.

Substitute Exercises

If you are not progressing in a specific area such as your chest training, then you may only need to substitute a couple of exercises. Doing so will stimulate the muscles in a new manner and employ different fibers than they have grown accustomed to. For instance, if you have been performing incline barbell presses for some time, try employing incline flies or presses with dumbbells. Another approach would be to substitute a free-weight exercise with a machine exercise. If you have been riding a stationary bike for a while, try another form of aerobic exercise such as running or swimming.

Evaluate Your Diet

It may be advantageous to look carefully at the food you have been consuming. People often underestimate just how important diet is to their exercise performance. If you have been eating mostly refined or high-fat foods rather than high-complex carbohydrate foods as suggested in the Revised American Diet, this could have a significant impact on your training energy and enthusiasm.

Take a Layoff

One sure-fire way to recover from either overtraining or a plateau in training progress is to take an all-out layoff from training. Usually a week or two is a sufficient interval. Use this time to evaluate your training. Make sure to get plenty of rest. It can be very inspiring to look through your training diary during this period. Examine your fitness goals to see how you might redefine them. The intention of a layoff is not to become sedentary – you should maintain some kind of activity. Try doing something different, such as bike riding, running or swimming, or even tai chi. Also, it is important to remember to maintain your flexibility. Although you may not be going to the gym, make a point of stretching each day.

Change Your Health Club

Though it may seem drastic to some, changing gyms is sometimes just the right trick. If you have been training at the same gym or health club for a while, you may have become accustomed to the same faces and equipment. I have trained all over this country and around the world, from Texas to Paris to South Africa. The energy has been different in each of these places. It's amazing what effect a different atmosphere, new people, and new equipment can have on your training. Some individuals maintain memberships at two or more gyms so that they have that variety available all the time.

Following are two advanced routines (A and B) that incorporate the pyramid, superset and triset principles presented in this section. The first routine incorporates supersets and trisets (those exercises with an asterisk before them), while the second routine employs pyramid sets.

	ADVANCED PROGRAM A Monday and Thursday	
	Sets	Reps
CHEST *Incline dumbbell press *Incline fly	3	8-12
Bench press	3	8-12
Cable cross-over	3	8-12
SHOULDERS *Seated dumbbell press *Dumbbell lateral raise *Rear-delt machine	3	8-12
TRICEPS *Cable tricep push-downs *Bench dip	3	8-12
Seated dumbbell tricep extension	3	8-12
ABDOMINALS *Hanging leg raise *Frog kick *Twisting crunch	3	15-25
CALVES *Standing heel raise *Seated heel raise	3	12-15

Aerobic activity: perform 30-45 minutes of aerobic activity.

*These exercises should be performed in supersets and trisets.

	ADVANCED PROGRAM A Tuesday and Friday	
	Sets	Reps
BACK		
*Seated cable row		
*Lat pull-downs	3	8-12
Dumbbell bent-over row	3	8-12
Back extension	3	12-15
BICEPS		
*Seated dumbbell curl		
*Dumbbell preacher curl	3	8-12
Concentration curl	3	8-12
FOREARMS		
*Reverse barbell curl		
*Barbell wrist curl	3	10-12

Aerobic activity: perform 30-45 minutes of aerobic activity.

*These exercises should be performed in supersets and trisets.

	ADVANCED PROGRAM A Wednesday and Saturday	
	Sets	Reps
LEGS		
*Lunge		
*Leg press	3	12-15
*Leg extension		
*Leg curl	3	12-15

Aerobic activity: perform 30-45 minutes of aerobic activity.

*These exercises should be performed in supersets and trisets.

ADVANCED PROGRAM B Monday and Thursday		
	Sets	Reps
CHEST		
Bench press	6	15, 12, 10, 8, 6, 4
Incline bench press	5	12, 10, 8, 6, 4
Flys	4	8-12
SHOULDERS		
Behind the neck press	5	12, 10, 8, 6, 4
Dumbbell lateral raises	4	8-12
Rear delt machine or bent-over lateral raise	4	8-12
TRICEPS		
Lying barbell tricep extension	5	12, 10, 8, 6, 4
Cable push-downs	4	8-12
Seated dumbbell tricep extension	4	8-12
CALVES		
Seated heel raise	5	12-15

ADVANCED PROGRAM B Tuesday and Friday		
	Sets	Reps
LEGS		
Leg press	6	15, 12, 10, 8, 6, 4
Leg extension	5	12, 10, 8, 6, 4
Leg curl	4	8-12
BACK		
Pull-up	4	12
Machine row	5	12, 10, 8, 6, 4
Dumbbell bent-over row	5	12, 10, 8, 6, 4
Back extension	3	12-15
BICEPS		
Standing barbell curl	5	12, 10, 8, 6, 4
Preacher curl	4	12, 10, 8, 6
Concentrate curl	4	8-12
ABDOMINALS		
Frog kick	3	15-25
Reverse crunch	3	15-25

Pyramid Sets

CHAPTER TWENTY-THREE

THE EXERCISES

We can now prove that large numbers of Americans
are dying from sitting on their behinds.
— Dr. Bruce B. Dan

Much of today's modern exercise equipment has a variety of possible settings for the user. For this reason it's important to examine a machine carefully before performing an exercise. It is likely that different adjustments have been made for the previous user. In order to have a safe and effective workout, it is important that you readjust the machine for your specific needs. This may include seat and foot pad height, and lever extension and starting points. Most modern equipment will have illustrations instructing you how to make these adjustments.

When performing any exercises lying on a bench, it is important to flatten your lower back. To achieve this, some individuals may have to place their feet on the bench with their knees bent, and to tilt the pelvis slightly.

LEG EXERCISES

SQUAT

Squats are highly effective for developing strength in the quadriceps. When done correctly, squats place primary stress on the quadricep muscles and secondary stress on the hamstrings or back of the thigh, buttocks (gluteal muscles), and the lower back (erector spinae).

First, load up a barbell with an appropriate weight. The bar should be on a squat rack and positioned so you can walk underneath. The bar should be lifted

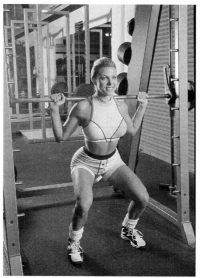

Squat: Smith Machine

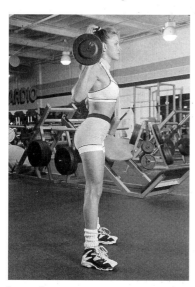

Squat: Start

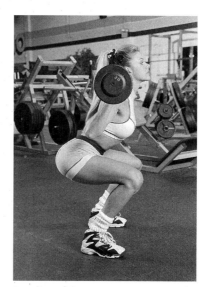

Finish

onto your upper back across your trapezius muscles. Stepping back from the rack, place your feet shoulders-width apart with your toes turned slightly outward. While keeping your back as straight as possible, inhale as you bend at the waist, then the knees, and descend into a squat position. Only squat to the point where your thighs are parallel to the floor. Exhale as you return to the start position.

The descending movement should be controlled and fluid; never drop or bounce into a squat position. Bouncing will put a great deal of stress on the tendons and ligaments that support the knee joint and could cause significant damage. It's important that you keep your torso as upright as possible and your eyes focused on the horizon while squatting. Also, avoid "bench squats," squats that are done with a bench placed beneath the thighs. Someone came up with the idea of squatting onto a bench to avoid passing the parallel point in the descent of the movement. However, it is easy to use the bench to push off from: the lifter may in fact perform a "touch-and-go" or bounce off the bench surface. Since the bench is a hard surface with little give, the weight resting on the upper back then causes compression in the spinal column and a squeezing effect on the intervertebral disks. For the sake of your back, stick with a squat rack or Smith machine for support.

LEG CURL

Leg curls strengthen the semitendinosus, semimembranosus, and bicep femoris muscles of the back of the thigh. Collectively these muscles are commonly referred to as the hamstrings.

Begin by lying facedown on the leg curl machine, making sure your knee joints are in alignment with the machine's axis of rotation. This will put the top of your knee just at the bench edge. You may need to adjust the roller pad so it meets your Achilles tendon. With your feet under the pad, begin to exhale and slowly pull the weight up with your hamstring muscles, bringing the roller of the lever to the back of your thighs. Lower the weight in a deliberate and controlled manner.

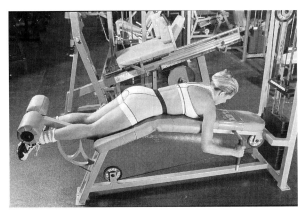

Leg curl: Start

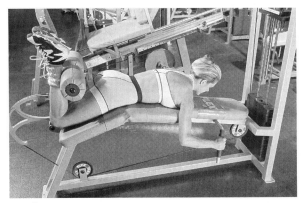

Finish

Seldom have I seen people perform this exercise properly. It requires great concentration, because the natural tendency is to lift one's hips from the machine to get the weight up. However, the hips must be kept against the bench for the exercise to be effective. There are a few machine manufacturers who have designed a leg-curling machine with a cambered bench to increase the isolation of the muscles and reduce the tendency to lift the hips. If you are fortunate enough to have one of these newer machines at your disposal, take advantage of it. Also, make a point of keeping your toes pointed throughout the movement. This will prevent the calf muscles (gastrocnemius and soleus) from becoming involved in the movement, and thus will isolate the hamstrings more effectively. Regardless of the machine you are using, I suggest that you keep your poundages to a minimum until you have mastered the movement.

LEG EXTENSION

Leg extensions isolate the quadriceps muscles and allow you to achieve a peak contraction. If the leg extension machine you use has an adjustable back, slide the back support up until it meets your back while keeping your knees in alignment with the machine's axis of rotation. After adjusting it to the right position, place your feet underneath the padded roller at the end of the lever. While grasping the side handles of the machine for support, exhale and slowly extend your legs in front of you until you have reached the top part of the movement. At this point hold your legs for a second or two, contracting the quadriceps muscles for a full peak contraction. Slowly lower the weight to the starting position.

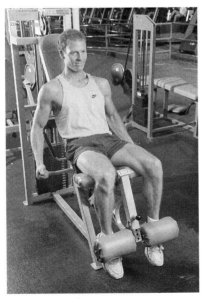

Leg extension: Start

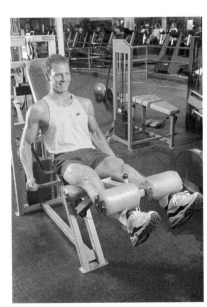

Finish

LEG PRESS

This exercise works the quadriceps, gluteal muscles, and hamstrings. Leg presses can be performed on a number of different machines, including a free-standing version, a Nautilus machine, and the Universal machine. I will describe the exercise as performed on a 45-degree-angle machine, since this seems to be both the most comfortable and popular version available.

Sit in the machine, resting your back on the padded backrest and making sure your hips are firm against the pad. Place your feet at shoulders-width on the pressing panel. On the outside of the machine there are tubular handles to grasp for support. These handles are also rotated outward to release the weight from its locked position. With the weight released, lower the weight slowly. Exhale as you return the weight to the top, extending your legs fully, remembering not to lock your knees.

As with squats, varying the placement of your feet will direct the stress to different areas in your thighs. A wider placement with your toes turned out will stress the inside of the thighs. Placing your feet closer together places more stress on the outside of the thigh.

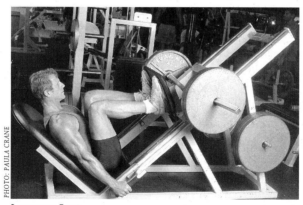

PHOTO: PAULA CRANE

Leg press: Start

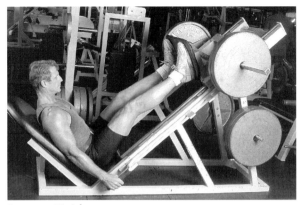

Leg press: Finish

LUNGE

The lunge is an excellent exercise that affects all of the muscles of the thigh as well as the gluteal muscles (buttocks). Stand erect with a barbell on your shoulders. Your feet should be placed a few inches apart, with your toes pointing straight

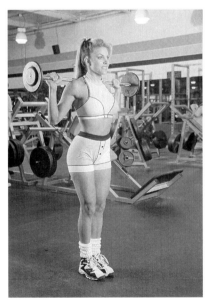

Lunge: Start

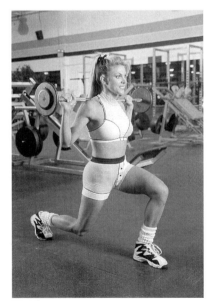

Finish

ahead. Take one step forward (either leg) and plant your foot flat on the floor. Bend the leg of the planted foot until your thigh is parallel with the floor (90 degrees). The length of your stride should allow you to maintain your shin in an upright position as you bend your knee. Be sure the knee of the forward leg is positioned directly over your foot and ankle. Exhale as you use your thigh muscle to straighten your leg and push yourself back to the starting position. Repeat the movement with your other leg for a single repetition. Lunges can also be performed using a Smith machine or with dumbbells in hand.

STANDING HEEL RAISE

The calf muscles, though small, are very strong and are capable of handling enormous poundages. In fact, you exercise them every day. Each time you take a step, you perform a partial calf raise using the resistance of your body weight.

The standing calf raise machine will place primary emphasis on the gastrocnemius muscles of the calves. The machine is very straightforward. Bend

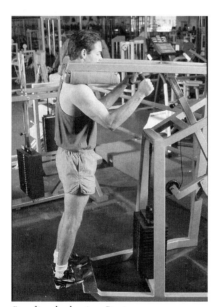
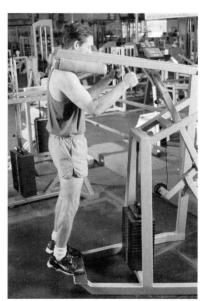

Standing heel raise: Start   Finish

down just enough to fit your shoulders under the shoulder pads and then step up onto the foot pad. Place your feet about shoulders-width apart. Grasp the tops of the shoulder pads for support while performing the exercise. It's important that you allow your heels to dip as far below the foot pad as possible for a complete stretch of the muscles. Then, raise yourself as high on the balls of your feet as you can, contracting your calf muscles at the top of the movement.

SEATED HEEL RAISE

This exercise will directly stress the soleus muscles of the calves.

After you are seated on the calf machine, adjust the knee pads so that they just slide over the tops of your knees when your feet are on the pedestal. Press on the balls of your feet until you can release the stop lever that has been securing the weight. Allow your heels to drop as deeply as possible. Then, raise your heels as high as you can, contracting the calf muscles at the top of the movement.

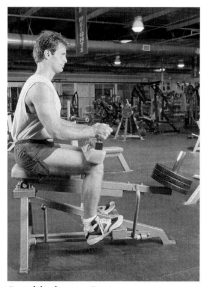
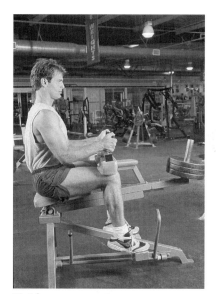

Seated heel raise: Start   Finish

CHEST EXERCISES

BENCH PRESS

This is one of the most essential exercises in any routine. The chief emphasis is placed on the chest; however, the shoulders and the tricep muscles benefit greatly from this movement.

Lie on a bench with your feet flat on the floor. Grasp the bar with at least a shoulders-width grip. Extend your arms and press the weight up and off the rack. Slowly lower the weight until the bar touches the middle of your chest (the weight should never be allowed to rest on the chest). Return to the top position without locking your elbows.

There are two harmful techniques that you must make a conscious effort to avoid. The first involves arching the back. NEVER arch your back while bench pressing. The result is a compression in the spine that could contribute to intervertebral disk injury. The second is bouncing the weight off your chest. When bouncing weight off your chest you are punishing a quite vulnerable part of your rib cage called the sternum. The poundages used in bench pressing are enough to crack the sternum if this technique is used.

You might be wondering why anybody would bounce the weight off their chest in the first place. It's really a cheating technique that coaxes the weight past a sticking point. The irony is that if you cheat past a weak point, you actually reduce the work load on the muscles. The less work those muscles do at that point, the weaker they will become! Remember to make a conscious effort to keep the movement as fluid as possible, and you won't develop weak points in the first place.

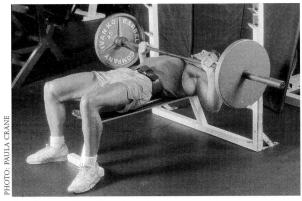

PHOTO: PAULA CRANE

Bench press: Start

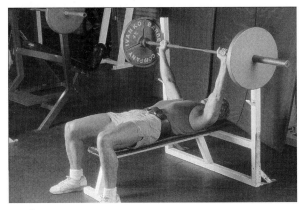

Finish

DUMBBELL BENCH PRESS

This movement is much like the regular bench press except that it is performed with dumbbells. The chest, shoulders, and triceps will benefit from this movement. As with all dumbbell movements initially, you may need to adjust to the independent arm action.

Lie back on an exercise bench with your feet either on the floor or on the bench. With dumbbells in hand, extend your arms above your chest without locking your elbows. Dumbbells should be facing end to end. Inhale as you lower the dumbbells in a controlled manner, allowing for a good pectoral stretch. Exhale as you return to the starting position.

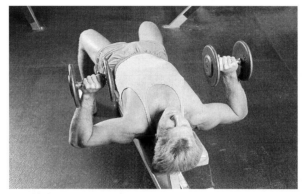

Dumbbell press: Start

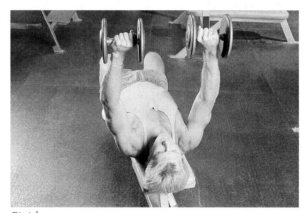

Finish

INCLINE BARBELL PRESS

This movement is much like the flat bench press except that it is performed at a 45-degree angle. At this angle, the stress will primarily be placed on the upper pectoral muscles and the shoulders (anterior deltoids).

Sit on the incline bench and lean back against the pad. Grasp the bar with a shoulders-width grip and your palms facing forward. On most incline racks, the weight will be resting just above your head. As you extend your arms, remove the weight from the rack and bring it forward until it is directly above your shoulders.

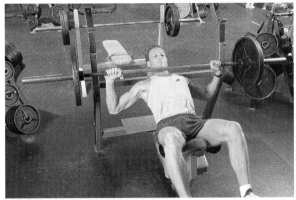

Incline barbell press: Start

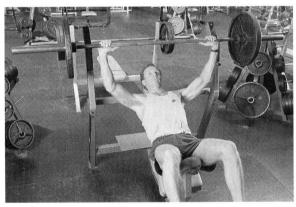

Finish

Slowly lower the weight until the bar reaches a point between the nipple line and the base of the neck. Exhale while pressing the weight back to the extended position.

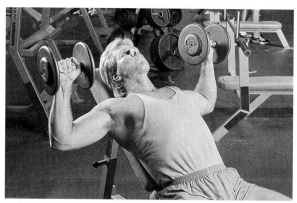

Incline dumbbell press: Start

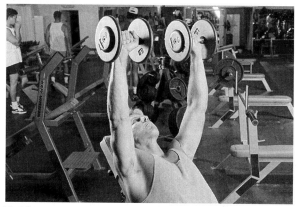

Finish

INCLINE DUMBBELL PRESS

This exercise involves the same movement as the incline barbell press, using dumbbells instead. By using dumbbells you will obtain a greater range of motion and a deeper stretch in the pectoral muscles. However, because dumbbells require a bit more coordinating, it's unlikely that you can handle the same poundage as you can using a barbell.

Because you are using dumbbells in this exercise, the weights will not be resting on a rack above you. It is important that you learn to get the dumbbells to and from the starting position in a safe manner.

Grasp a pair of dumbbells and sit on the incline bench. Place the dumbbells on end and on your thighs, just above your knees. While leaning back on the bench, in one fluid movement, push one foot off the ground with your toes. As you raise your knee toward your body, you will be able to transfer the weight safely from your knee to your upper chest. Then in the same manner, transfer the other dumbbell from the other knee to your upper chest. With both dumbbells at your upper chest, press up until your arms are extended fully overhead. In order to maintain proper form, imagine that the dumbbells are connected by a bar, just like a barbell. Lower the weight at the same point you would a barbell until you have achieved a deep stretch. Return the weight to the top position.

Some people who perform this movement have an unconscious tendency to rotate the wrists until they are facing one another rather than straight ahead. As a result, the movement is changed to something quite similar to a fly, as opposed to a press. Maintaining the mental image of a barbell in your hands should keep you from making this mistake, since the described wrist rotation is impossible with a barbell.

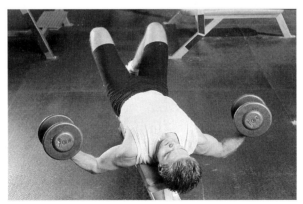

Fly: Start

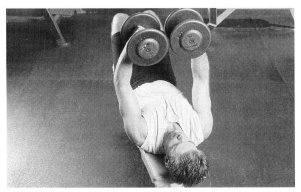
Fly: Finish

DUMBBELL FLY

The fly is a wonderful movement for shaping and strengthening the pectoral muscles. The fly is an isolation exercise that stresses the inner and outer edges of the muscles.

As with dumbbell incline presses, it is important that you make a conscious effort to watch for wrist rotation in this movement. The fly movement is actually like giving someone a big hug, so make sure you don't start performing dumbbell presses.

Grasp a pair of dumbbells and lie back on an exercise bench. Extend your arms above you. Keeping your elbows slightly flexed, slowly lower the weight, your arms opening into a wide arc as you go. Allow gravity to pull that arc and give you a deep stretch in the chest. While maintaining the arc, pull with your chest, bringing your arms back to the starting point. Contract the pectoral muscles tightly. Be sure to keep the dumbbells moving on a plane even with your shoulders.

INCLINE DUMBBELL FLY

This movement is much the same as dumbbell flies except that it is performed at an incline. Choose an exercise bench that allows you to adjust its incline to approximately 45 degrees. Perform the fly movement described above, making sure to avoid wrist rotation.

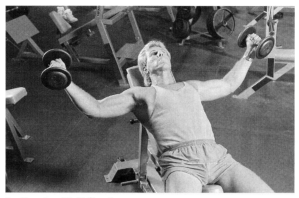

Incline dumbbell fly: Start

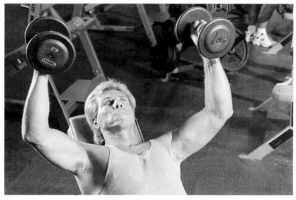

Near finish

CABLE CROSSOVER

Cable crossovers are excellent for stressing the inner and outer areas of the pectoral region.

While standing, center yourself between the two cable stations. Grasp one pulley handle and then the other. Take a step forward and bend slightly at the waist. Slowly bring the cables downward, your arms moving in a semicircle until your hands cross past one another. Squeeze the pectoral muscles tightly before returning to the starting position. A variation includes bending more at the waist. As your torso becomes more parallel to the floor, the emphasis of the exercise will be directed toward the upper pectoral muscles. A more upright stance directs the emphasis to the lower pectoral region.

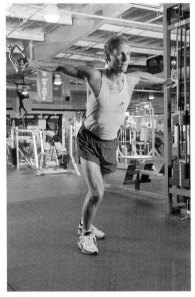 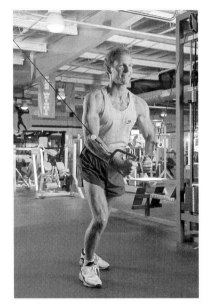

Cable Crossover: Start   Finish

PEC-DECK FLY

This exercise is much like the regular fly except that it is done in an upright position.

Pec-deck machines vary in the number of adjustments that can be made by the user. In most cases you should be able to adjust the height of the seat. On one type of machine this is done by spinning the seat; another incorporates a spring-loaded selector pin. At proper height, your arms should be in line with your chest. Some of the newer machines will allow you to adjust the length of the machine levers, using the same type of selector pin.

After making your adjustments, sit in the machine. Place either forearm behind the pad. Then, while pulling the first arm with you, turn your torso toward the other pad and slip your forearm behind it. Allow the weight to pull your arms back for a complete stretch of the pectoral muscles. Slowly bring your arms together

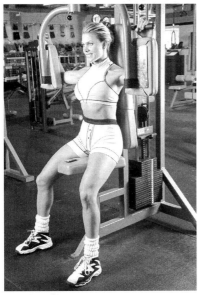 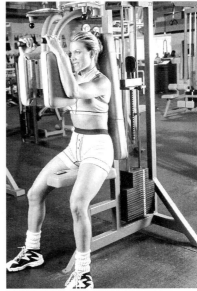

Pec-deck fly: Start   Finish

until the pads touch. Contract your chest muscles tightly before returning to the starting position. Make sure not to move your head or your hips away from the bench. They should remain firm against the pad at all times.

MACHINE CHEST PRESS

Although there is a wide variety of chest press machines available, their design is very similar. The most important adjustment you need to make is the seat height. Adjust the seat position so that the handles of the pressing lever meet at the nipple line. If the machine has a foot pedal, press it to bring the lever handles forward.

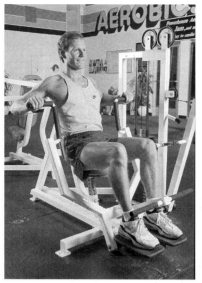 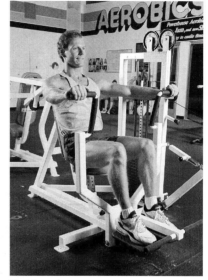

Machine chest press: Start   Finish

Grasp the handles and exhale as you press forward, without locking your elbows. Return to the starting position.

SHOULDER EXERCISES

BEHIND-THE-NECK PRESS

This is an old standby movement that is fantastic for developing upper-body strength. The chief emphasis is on the shoulders (specifically the anterior head of the deltoid muscles), while secondary emphasis is on the triceps and upper-back muscles.

Although this exercise can be performed either standing or seated, the seated version is much safer.

Grasp a barbell from a rack behind you and assume a wider-than-shoulders-width grip. From a seated position, slowly lower the barbell behind your neck. Exhaling, press the bar up. Slowly return the weight to the beginning position.

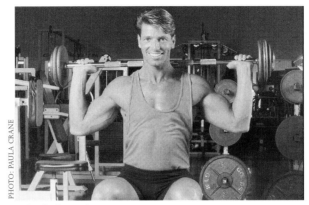

PHOTO: PAULA CRANE

Behind-the-neck press: Start

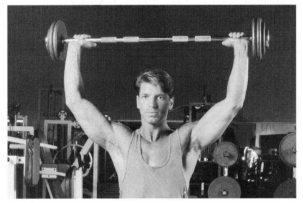

Finish

This movement can be duplicated using a Smith machine, which has a barbell permanently installed within it. The bar moves vertically within two tracks. At various points along the track the bar can be "locked out," and the exerciser can dismount the machine. The advantage of the Smith machine is that the bar is already in an elevated position and need not be hoisted from the floor. Also, the bar can be locked out at any time, should the exerciser feel too fatigued to complete a repetition.

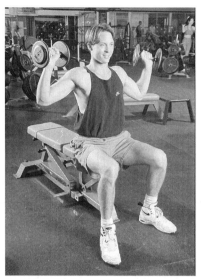
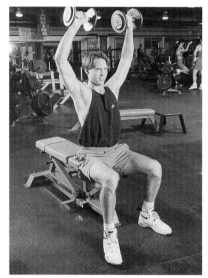

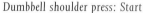
Dumbbell shoulder press: Start   Finish

SEATED DUMBBELL SHOULDER PRESS

This is much like the behind-the-neck press. Dumbbell presses primarily stress the anterior head of the deltoid and the tricep muscles.

With dumbbells in hand, sit on the end of an exercise bench. You can utilize a similar movement to that used to get the dumbbells to your chest when performing dumbbell incline presses. Place the dumbbells on your knees and alternately push them up to your shoulders. Slowly press the dumbbells upward, palms out, until just before your elbows lock. Lower the weight to your shoulders and repeat.

DUMBBELL LATERAL RAISE

Lateral raises work the lateral head of the deltoid muscles and are excellent for adding shape to the shoulders.

Grasp a pair of dumbbells. Your feet should be about shoulders-width apart. While bending slightly forward at the waist, raise the dumbbells out to your sides in semicircles until they are slightly above shoulder level. Then, in a controlled manner, lower the dumbbells along the same arc, returning to the starting position.

Chances are that if you see people swinging dumbbells in this movement, they are using too heavy a set of dumbbells. This is an isolation exercise and is very demanding of the deltoid muscles. For this reason, it is not necessary to use a lot

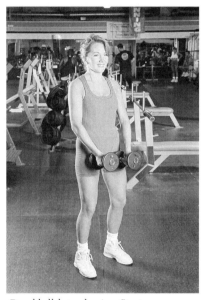 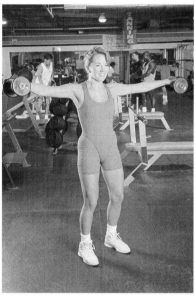

Dumbbell lateral raise: Start   *Finish*

of weight if you employ strict form. Experienced lifters know how to make a set of 15-pound dumbbells feel like a set of 30s through the use of strict form. So go after the feeling, not the numbers imprinted on the dumbbells.

DUMBBELL FRONTAL RAISE

This exercise strongly stresses the anterior head of the deltoid muscles. Grasp a pair of dumbbells. While standing, feet shoulders-width apart, elbows slightly bent, slowly raise one dumbbell in a semicircular arc in front of you to a point

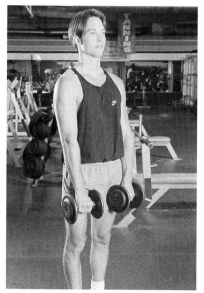 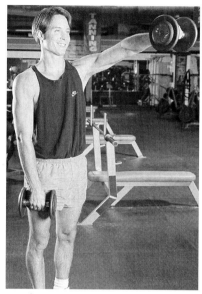

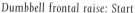
Dumbbell frontal raise: Start   Finish

just above shoulder level. Slowly lower the dumbbell to the starting position and then repeat the movement with your other arm, continuing to alternate between arms. Make sure not to rock or swing the weight up.

BENT-OVER LATERAL RAISE

This exercise is for developing strength in the posterior (rear) head of the deltoid muscles, and places secondary stress on the muscles of the upper back. This movement can also be performed on an upright rear-deltoid machine.

Grasp a pair of dumbbells and sit on the end of an exercise bench. Bend over at the waist until your torso is parallel to the floor, making sure to keep your back straight. Your arms should be hanging to the ground and bent slightly, with your palms facing inward. Slowly raise the dumbbells in semicircular arcs to the sides of your torso until they reach a point slightly above your shoulders. Return the dumbbells in the same arc to the beginning position.

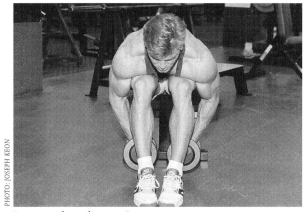

PHOTO: JOSEPH KEON

Bent-over lateral raise: Start

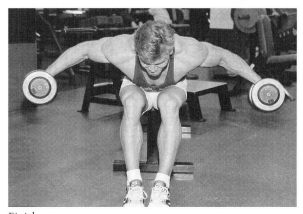

Finish

CABLE LATERAL RAISE

This isolation exercise affects the anterior and lateral heads of the deltoid muscles.

Station yourself about two feet from the floor pulley mechanism. Your feet should be about shoulders-width apart. Grasp the pulley handle with one hand. Keeping your back straight, bend forward slightly at the waist. Your other hand can be placed on your hip or used to grasp the pulley station for support.

With your arm slightly bent, raise the handle, pulling the cable across your body to a point just above the shoulder. Slowly lower the weight to the starting position. Repeat the same movement for the other side.

A variation is to perform this exercise with the cable running diagonally across the back of the body.

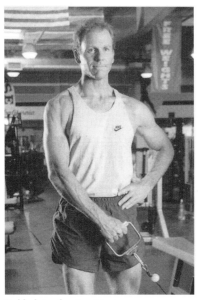
Cable lateral raise: Start

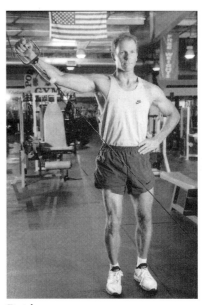
Finish

REAR-DELT MACHINE

The rear-delt machine is usually a two-function machine, allowing one to perform both upright flies for the chest as well as exercise the rear deltoids.

The movement is very much the same as the bent-over lateral raise except that it is done in an upright position. This position allows for greater isolation of the working muscle (rear deltoid), while placing secondary stress on the muscles of the upper back and the medial head of the deltoid muscles.

Sit on the machine with your torso erect and your chest and hips firmly against the pad. Grasp the handles and, using your rear deltoid muscles, pull your arms back in an arcing fashion. Return to the starting position and repeat.

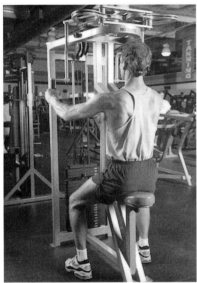
Rear-delt machine: Start

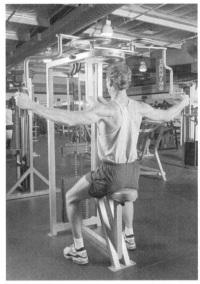
Finish

BACK EXERCISES

PULL-UP

Pull-ups are excellent for strengthening and developing the entire back. You probably were asked to perform 10 of these in your high school physical education course at one time or another. In my class, there were few who could perform more than three. It amazed me because even the biggest, toughest guys couldn't pull their own body weight up more than a few times. If you have never performed a pull-up, the movement may seem nearly impossible at first. However, in a short time you will be performing sets of them.

Take a wide, overhand grip on the pull-up bar. Bend your knees, both for stability and ground clearance. Pull yourself up until your chin is above the bar, and then lower yourself completely for a full stretch of the latissimus muscles. Alternatives include pull-ups to the rear, a palms-in grip, which places more emphasis on the bicep muscles, and variations in grip width.

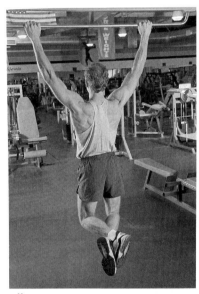 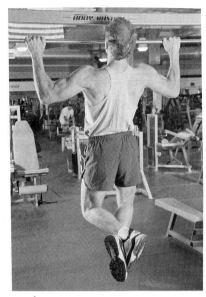

Pull-up: Start   Finish

For those who have not yet developed the strength to lift their body, pull-ups can be performed on either a Gravitron machine or Cybex pull-up/dip assist station. Both of these popular devices can be adjusted to compensate for a portion of your body weight, thus allowing you to perform the full range of movement.

LAT PULL-DOWN

Pull-downs are a great exercise for overall back strength and development.

Sit down and wedge your knees under the restraining pad of the machine. Grasp the pull-down bar with an overhand grip, placing your hands slightly wider than shoulders-width apart. Exhale as you slowly pull the bar down until it touches your upper chest. Contract the muscles of your back fully and return the bar to the beginning point. Make sure to extend your arms fully with each rep to ensure a full range of motion.

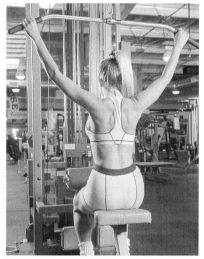

Lat pull-down: Start

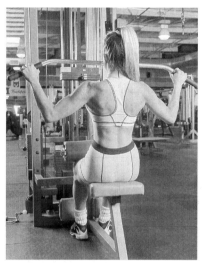

Finish

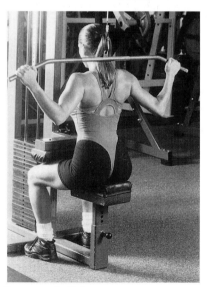

Variation: Pull-down to rear

A variation of this exercise is to pull the bar to your upper back. Doing so may be difficult and could be dangerous for those who have a limited range of movement.

SEATED CABLE ROW

When it comes to back exercises, this rowing movement seems to be a favorite. The movement works the entire back, and places secondary emphasis on the biceps, brachialis, and posterior deltoids.

Sit on the rowing machine bench and place your feet on the restraining bar in front. Grasp the cable handle and sit nearly erect, arms extended. Keeping your

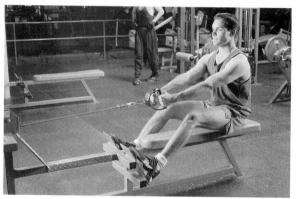

Seated cable row: Start

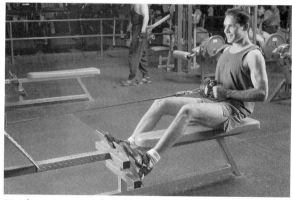

Finish

back straight, exhale as you pull the handle into your abdominal region. Extend your arms slowly, leaning slightly forward from the waist. Make sure to squeeze your shoulders at the top part of the movement so as to ensure a complete contraction of the lat muscles.

DUMBBELL BENT-OVER ROW

While bending forward at the waist, your back parallel to the floor, place one hand and knee on the side of an exercise bench for support. Bending your opposite knee slightly, and rotating your torso slightly, grasp the dumbbell. Slowly pull the dumbbell up to the side of your torso. Then, lower the dumbbell slowly for a deep stretch, this time rotating your torso toward the dumbbell as you do so. Repeat

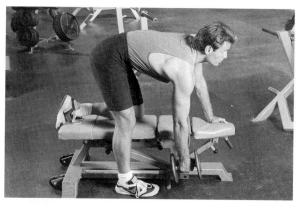

Dumbbell bent-over row: *Start*

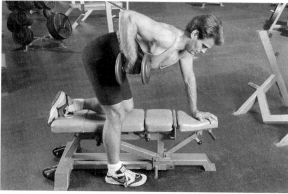

Finish

for the suggested number of repetitions. Then switch arms, performing the same number of reps for the other side to make a complete set.

BACK EXTENSION

Back extensions are another exercise that allows for a peak contraction. The primary emphasis is placed on the erector spinae muscles of the lumbar (lower) region of the back. Secondary stress is placed on the hamstrings and the gluteal muscles.

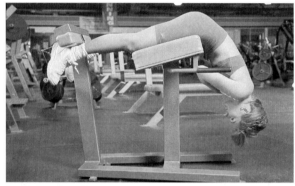

Back extension: Start

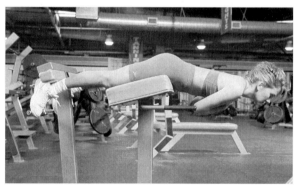

Finish

Situate yourself between the two pads of the back extension station. You should be facing the larger of the two pads. On the sides of this pad are support handles. Grasp these handles and lower your hips to just beyond the pad. Permit your legs to come up behind you and wedge the backs of your ankles under the smaller, rear pad. Slide forward until your torso can hang down from your hips. Interlock your hands behind your head or cross them in front of your chest. As you exhale, slowly raise your torso until both torso and legs are in line with one another. Make sure to focus on using just the lower back muscles to lift your torso, and avoid any swinging or rhythmic movement.

MACHINE ROW

Machine rows strengthen the entire back. Adjust the seat to the appropriate height and be seated. Then, adjust the chest support pad so that, when your arms are fully extended, the plates do not touch the weight stack. This will allow for a

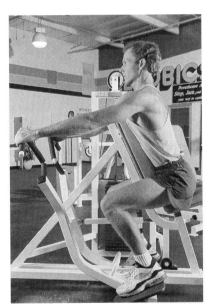

Machine row: Start

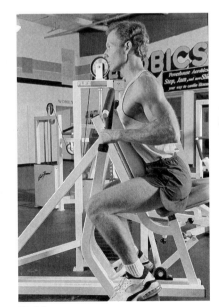

Finish

full range of motion. Exhale as you pull the handles back in a smooth rowing motion. Return to the starting position and repeat.

DUMBBELL SHRUG

The shrug is an isolation exercise that focuses on the trapezius muscles of the upper back.

Grasp a pair of dumbbells. Concentrating on the trapezius muscles, slowly shrug your shoulders upward. Think of trying to touch your ears with your shoulders. Your arms should remain straight and not be involved in the lift, except to hold the weight. At the top of the movement, squeeze the trapezius muscles tightly, then lower the weight, allowing your shoulders to sag deeply. A variation is to perform shrugs with a barbell.

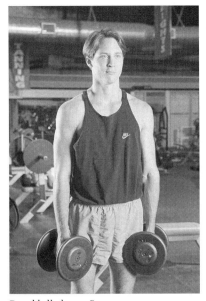

Dumbbell shrug: Start

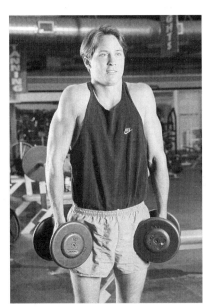

Finish

BICEP EXERCISES

STANDING BARBELL CURL

This is the old standby bicep exercise. Barbell curls work the entire bicep muscle. Secondary stress is placed on the flexor muscles of the forearm. With your

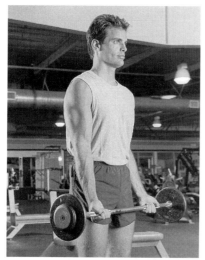

Barbell curl: Start

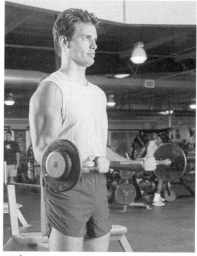

Mid-point

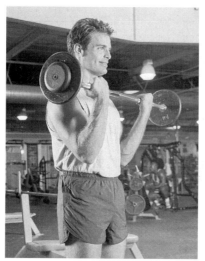

Finish

feet at a medium stance, grasp a barbell with a shoulders-width, underhand grip. Allow the bar to hang from your fully extended arms. While keeping your back erect, slowly curl the bar up to just below your chin. Lower the bar in a controlled manner. This exercise can also be performed with an E-Z curl bar, which you may find more comfortable.

PREACHER BENCH CURL

Preacher bench curls effectively isolate the bicep muscles. Grasp a barbell with an underhand grip. Your hands should be at shoulders-width. With the top of the

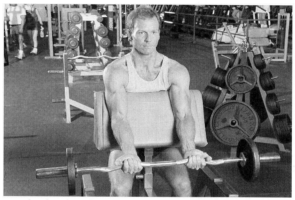

Preacher bench curl: Start

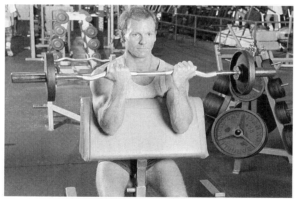

Finish

preacher bench wedged under your arms, extend your arms fully. From the fully extended position, curl the weight up to the top position, fully contracting the bicep muscles.

Try to avoid leaning back when performing this exercise. Ideally, you should lean forward a bit to ensure maximum isolation of the working muscle. Preacher bench curls can be performed with a barbell, cables, or dumbbells.

SEATED DUMBBELL CURL

This exercise can be performed with both dumbbells simultaneously or alternately. Since the exercise is performed while seated, there is less of a tendency to "cheat" the weight up.

Grasp two dumbbells and sit on the end of an exercise bench. Allow both arms to hang at your sides. Exhale as you slowly curl the weight up toward your frontal deltoids. At the top portion of the movement, squeeze the biceps and then lower the weight to the starting position.

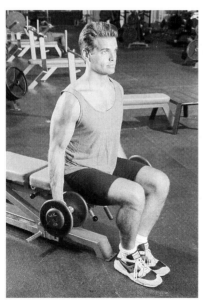
Seated dumbbell curl: Start

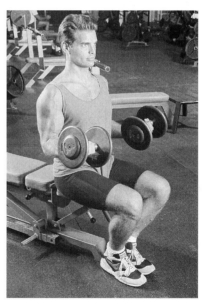
Near finish

Cable curls can be performed either with both arms using a short bar attachment, or with one arm at a time using a loop-shaped handle. One can achieve greater isolation performing the exercise one arm at a time.

Standing about one-and-a-half to two feet from the base of the cable apparatus, grasp the cable handle with an underhand grip, keeping your upper arm close to your torso. Begin the movement with your arm fully extended. Then curl the weight up, much as you would while performing barbell curls, bringing the handle toward your frontal deltoid. Lower the weight in a controlled fashion and repeat the movement for the required number of reps.

I suggest that you experiment with one-arm cable curls, as well. You will be able to use a variety of postures with the one-arm cable handle and, consequently, vary the effect on your biceps significantly.

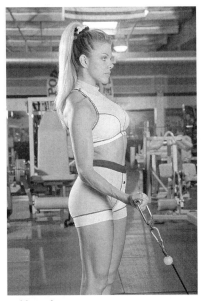

Cable curl: Start

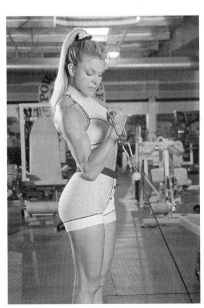

Finish

CONCENTRATION CURL

Concentration curls allow for strict isolation of the biceps as well as a peak contraction.

Grasp a dumbbell and sit on the end of an exercise bench. With your feet spread apart, bend over and place the elbow of the working arm against the inside of the thigh of the same side. To support your torso, grasp your other knee with your free hand. Beginning with your arm fully extended, slowly curl the weight up, keeping the dumbbell aligned with the bicep, contracting the bicep fully at the top. Slowly lower the dumbbell for a full stretch in the bicep. Repeat for suggested number of reps.

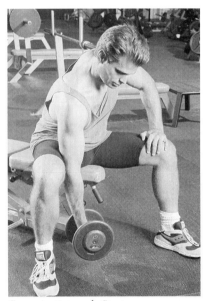

Concentration curl: Start

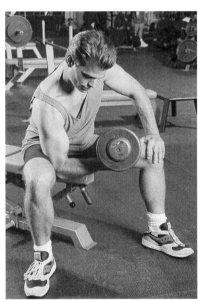

Finish

TRICEP EXERCISES

SEATED DUMBBELL TRICEP EXTENSION

This exercise allows for a deep stretch in the tricep and places the greatest stress on the inner head of the three-headed tricep muscle.

Grasp a dumbbell and sit on the end of an exercise bench. Extend your arm overhead. Slowly lower the dumbbell behind your neck, allowing for a deep stretch at the bottom part of the movement. Exhale as you return the dumbbell to the extended position. Make sure not to allow the weight to bounce into the down position.

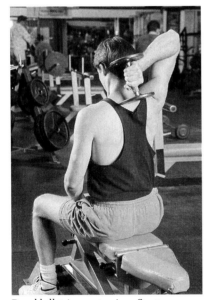
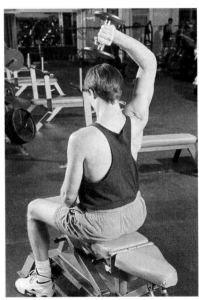

Dumbbell tricep extension: Start   Near finish

LYING BARBELL TRICEP EXTENSION

This exercise is a mainstay for overall tricep development. Lie on a bench. Beginning with a narrow grip and the bar extended overhead, lower the bar about halfway behind your head. Return the bar to the extended position. Make sure to keep the upper arms stationary, and elbows in toward the midline of the body. Be careful not to bump your head. Avoid lowering the bar to your forehead as this may cause discomfort in the elbow joint.

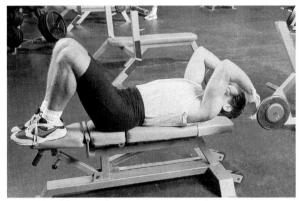

Barbell tricep extension: Start

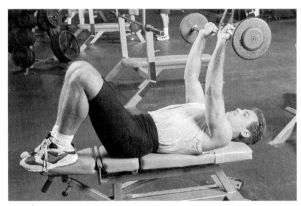

Finish

TRICEP PUSH-DOWN

Push-downs work the entire tricep while placing particular stress on the outer head of the muscle.

Place yourself about six inches from the pulley station. Take a narrow grip on the cable crossbar, your palms facing the floor. While keeping your elbows at your sides, press the bar down until just before your elbows lock out. Contract the tricep muscles fully and raise the crossbar to the starting point. Variations include using V-shaped bars and rope handle attachments.

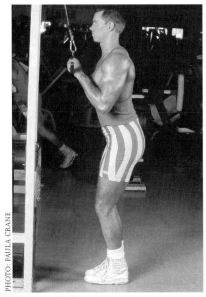 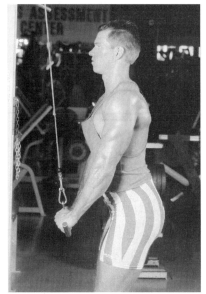

PHOTO: PAULA CRANE

Tricep push-down: Start   Finish

DUMBBELL KICKBACK

This exercise provides a peak contraction in the tricep muscles.

Grasp a dumbbell in one hand and lean over, resting your hand on either the end of an exercise bench or a dumbbell rack. Your torso should be parallel to the floor. Hold your exercising arm against your torso and bend at the elbow, allowing your forearm to drop so it is perpendicular to the floor. Exhale as you slowly straighten your arm out behind you. At the top of the movement contract your tricep muscles fully. Lower the weight to the starting position and repeat the movement. Perform the same movement for the other arm. This exercise can also be done using a cable and pulley station.

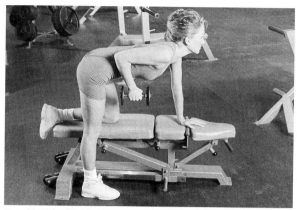

Dumbbell kickback: Start

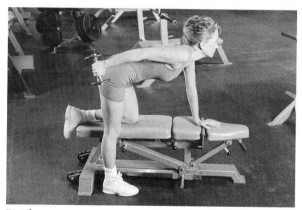

Finish

PARALLEL BAR DIP

Dips condition the triceps, pectoral muscles, and the frontal deltoids.

Climb onto a dipping station apparatus. Grasp the bars with your palms facing each other. Bend your knees, keeping your elbows at your sides, and lower yourself only to the point where your arms are bent at a 90-degree angle. As you exhale, return to the top of the movement without locking your elbows.

In order to keep the primary stress on the triceps, it is important that you keep your torso as upright as possible throughout the movement. In order to place more emphasis on the pectoral muscles, lean your torso forward throughout the movement and allow your elbows to move away from the sides of your torso. As you gain strength in this movement, you can either use a weight belt, or clutch a

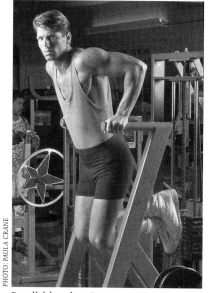

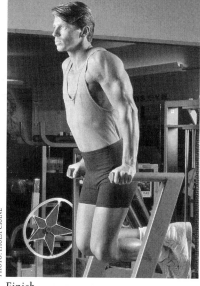

Parallel bar dip: Start   *Finish*

dumbbell between your feet during the movement. Dips can also be performed on a Gravitron or Cybex pull-up/dip assist station.

ABDOMINAL EXERCISES

CRUNCH

The crunch is an isolation exercise that effectively develops the entire abdominal region. As previously mentioned, crunches are especially safe for anyone with a lower-back condition.

Lie on your back with your knees bent, and rest your calves over an exercise bench. You should be close enough to the bench so that your knees are directly over your hips. Interlace your fingers behind your neck at the base of the skull.

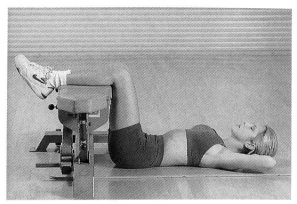

Crunch: *Start*

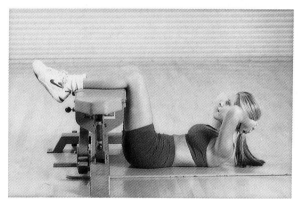

Finish

Using your abdominal muscles, slowly raise your shoulders, head, and neck from the floor, exhaling as you go. Return to the start position slowly, keeping your abdominal muscles contracted.

HANGING LEG RAISE

This exercise will stress the entire abdominal region with particular stress placed on the lower area.

Grasp a pull-up bar with a medium-width, overhand grip. Bend your knees to remove the curve in your back. From this point, using your abdominals, pull your knees up to your chest. Slowly lower your legs to the starting position. There is a tendency to swing the body during this movement. Try to avoid this. If you have a training partner, ask him or her to press against your lower back for stability.

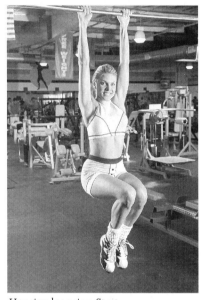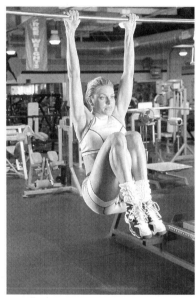

Hanging leg raise: Start   Finish

BENT-KNEE SIT-UP

This exercise can be performed on a sit-up board or on the floor. The board will usually include a strap under which you can secure your feet. On the floor you may wish to have a training partner hold your feet secure. Lie on your back with your knees bent, feet on the floor. With your hands interlaced behind your head, use your abdominal muscles to lift your torso toward your chest. Return to the starting position and repeat.

Some individuals feel more stress in their hip flexor muscles (the pelvic region) than their abdominals. Others are able to effectively isolate the abdominals. Experiment and see what works for you. You may prefer the crunch to the bent-knee sit-up. If you have any sort of lower-back condition it is best for you to choose another exercise, such as the crunch.

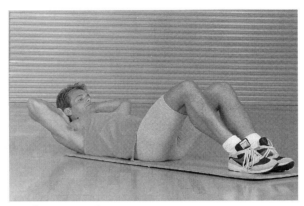

Bent-knee sit-up: Start

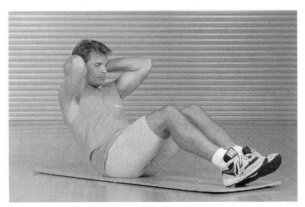

Finish

BICYCLE

Bicycles are similar to the twisting crunch except for the added dimension of leg movement. Lie on your back with your knees bent, feet on the floor. Simultaneously, lift and twist your right shoulder while bringing your left knee forward. Your right elbow and left knee should meet. Extend your left leg while

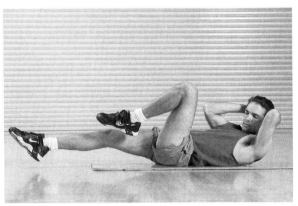
Bicycle: Start

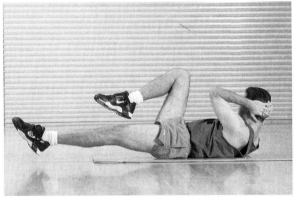
Finish

bringing the right knee and left elbow in contact. Continue this alternation in a fluid manner while keeping your abdominals contracted.

FROG KICK

Sit on the end of an exercise bench. Grasp the sides of the bench for support. Lean back and extend your legs in front of you. Bend your legs and bring your knees up toward your chest. At the top of the movement contract your abdominals tightly. Return to the starting position, and repeat.

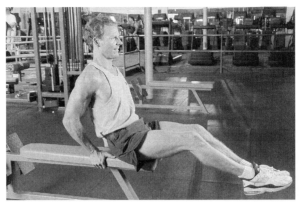

Frog kick: Start

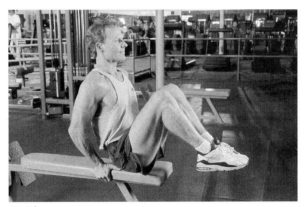

Finish

LEG PULL-IN

This exercise primarily affects the lower abdominals. Lie on a floor, placing your hands just underneath your lower buttocks, with your palms facing the floor. Bend your knees and pull your legs in so that the tops of your thighs are touching your abdomen. Simultaneously, tuck in your chin as your knees come forward. Extend your legs again to the starting position, and repeat.

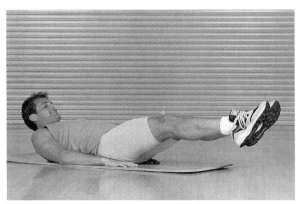

Leg pull-in: Start

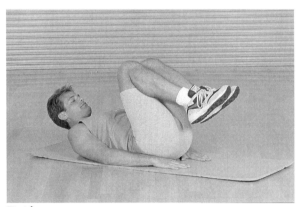

Finish

TWISTING CRUNCH

The twisting crunch is similar to the regular crunch, but at the top of the movement you move your opposite elbow across your body. As the repetitions proceed, alternate elbows. This exercise will shift the emphasis to the oblique muscles, those which cover the lower eight ribs.

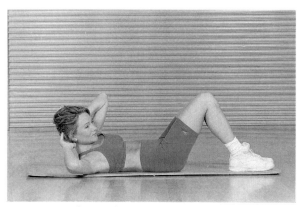

Twisting crunch: Finish

REVERSE CRUNCH

Lie on your back at the foot of an exercise bench or other apparatus that you can grasp for support. After grasping the support, bend your knees to a 90-degree angle. Focusing on your abdominals, bring your thighs toward your chest, slightly lifting your pelvis from the floor as you do so. In a controlled manner, return your legs to the 90-degree angle starting position. Be sure not to rest your feet on the ground.

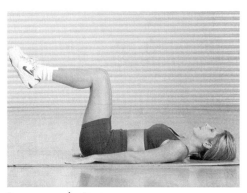

Reverse crunch: Start

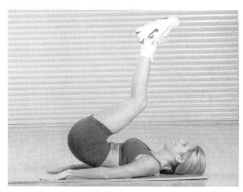

Finish

FOREARM EXERCISES

WRIST CURL

Wrist curls develop the powerful flexor muscles of the forearm.

Grasp a barbell with a narrow-width, underhand grip and rest the backs of your wrists and forearms on the end of a bench. Begin with the bar hanging in your fingers. Then, slowly curl your fingers, making a fist until the forearm muscles are fully contracted. Lower the weight until it hangs from your fingers again.

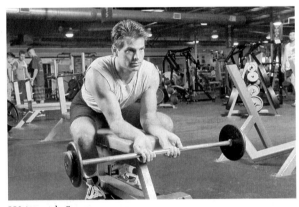

Wrist curl: Start

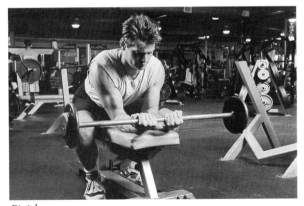

Finish

Reverse curls stress the brachialis and brachioradialis muscles of the outside of the bicep and forearm.

This movement is much like performing a barbell curl for the biceps. However, with reverse curls, a reverse or overhand grip is used. Grasp the bar with a medium-width grip. Allow the barbell to hang against your thighs. With your elbows pinned close to your torso, curl the weight up in a semicircular arc toward your chin. Return the weight to the starting position. Make sure to keep your upper body still throughout this movement.

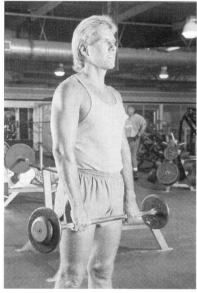

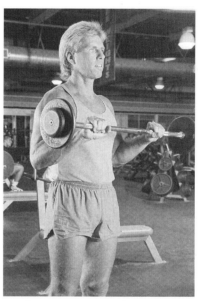

Barbell reverse curl: Start   Finish

Book
Three

The Mind-Body Connection

CHAPTER TWENTY-FOUR

THE MIND-BODY CONNECTION

For every thought supported by feeling, there is a muscle change.
Primary muscle patterns being the biological heritage of man,
man's whole body records his emotional thinking.
—Mabel Ellsworth

So far we have seen that, in an effort to maintain excellent health, we must work toward muscular strength and flexibility, aerobic conditioning, and healthy nutrition. To complete the Whole Health Equation presented at the beginning of this book, there is one final area we must address: the mind. Today it is increasingly clear that our physical health and well-being are contingent not only on a well-conditioned body, but on a mind that has been properly focused and conditioned as well.

For centuries, approaches to medical treatment reflected the belief that mind, body, and soul were inseparable. During the mid-seventeenth century, however, a renewed emphasis on the scientific method, resulting in a fundamental change in this philosophy, was brought about by the leading thinkers of the time. Isaac Newton saw the universe as a massive machine, one that could be broken down into separate parts composed of tangible matter. Newton's views became highly influential and directed thinking in a linear and geometrical direction. Consequently, ideas about maintaining human health became focused on viewing the body as a machine or robot composed of "units," each operating individually and with no relationship to the others. When illness arose, it was viewed as something that originated in the material (or bodily) realm and therefore could have no relationship to the mind.

THE WHOLISTIC VIEW

Although some people still regard the mind and the body as two independent entities, a new perspective has emerged. This perspective was first popularized by Albert Einstein and later carried on by many modern physicists such as David Bohm and Fritjof Capra. With this contemporary perspective, often referred to as *systemic* or *wholistic*, we can see clearly that the body and all of its various organs and tissues (including the mind) are actually highly interactional. We can no longer focus on a single part of the body without considering its relationship to the whole, nor can we expect to achieve and maintain a high degree of health without addressing the entire interdependent system.

CHAPTER TWENTY-FIVE

STRESS

To get the body in tone, get the mind in tune.
—Zachary T. Bercovitz, M.D.

Illnesses that were once thought to stem solely from the body may be more accurately seen as a physical manifestation of something mental, that is, our state of mind and emotions. It is becoming increasingly clear that our beliefs, thoughts, and feelings can significantly influence our physical health and performance.

One of the most serious consequences of mind-body interplay seen today (and one of our greatest health concerns) is something we've come to refer to as stress. While most of us have at some time heard that stress is unhealthy, few people understand why this is so. What is stress anyway? And what is it doing other than "wearing us down" or making us feel tired?

In this chapter, we will first look closely at exactly what stress is and also examine some of its causes. We will then explore ways to prevent stress from developing, to diffuse it should it occur, and learn to create a greater balance in the relationship between mind and body.

WHAT IS STRESS?

Dr. Hans Selye, often referred to as the "father of stress," popularized the term in the 1950s. Selye differentiated between *stress*, which he defined as "the nonspecific response of the organism to any pressure or demand," and the *stressor*, which he defined as "the stimulus, either an internal or external occurrence or event which produces the stress response." However, as we will see, it is important to remember that so-called stressors only have the potential to produce stress. Not all stressors produce stress in every individual. What is most important is our perception of the events in our lives. For example, two people are driving home in commute traffic on the same crowded freeway. While the situation has the potential to produce stress, one of these two people copes effectively with the commute, experiencing little or no stress, while the other is overwhelmed by the experience and undergoes severe emotional and physical distress. The same stressor is present for both people, yet only one experiences stress.

The stressors that we most commonly experience are associated with such events as accidents, illness, fights, divorce, work deadlines, presentations, exams, financial burdens, and, of course, rush-hour traffic. Stressors, when responded to inappropriately, can take a significant toll on our health, leading to headaches, insomnia, ulcers, adrenal failure, high blood pressure, stroke, and heart attack. Simply put, stress can kill. Chronic stress has the effect of suppressing the function of the immune system, resulting in our being significantly more susceptible to illness and disease. In fact, current estimates are that nearly 75 percent of all visits to physicians are the result of a stress-related illness.

To understand how a stressful experience can have such an influence on our health, it is necessary to examine a human reaction known as the fight or flight response.

THE FIGHT OR FLIGHT RESPONSE

The fight or flight response includes a series of physiological changes that take place in response to a perceived threat. This physiological process evolved over millions of years and now is a component of our genetic makeup. It is the legacy of the "survival of the fittest." For our ancient ancestor, the caveman, fight or flight was a life-saver. For people today, this primitive physiological response can have grave consequences.

Consider the ancient cave dweller. At all times he was at risk of attack by wild animals. Suppose he was sitting at his fire, when suddenly a saber-toothed tiger entered his cave. In split-second timing, the cave dweller would need to make a decision about how he would handle this uninvited guest. Essentially he had two choices: either stay and fight, or take flight and get out of the animal's way. For either choice, the cave-dweller's body would be prepared for action by way of his autonomic nervous system (ANS). The autonomic portion of the nervous system regulates internal states such as functions of the heart, blood pressure, and digestion. The ANS has two branches: the sympathetic and the parasympathetic. It is the sympathetic portion, the branch responsible for arousal, that stimulates the fight or flight response. In doing so, it releases powerful hormones that lead to a state of heightened arousal. Several powerful changes occur during the fight or flight response. They include:

- Dilation of the pupils to increase visual sensitivity

- Dilation of the bronchioles in the lungs and increased rate of breathing to allow more oxygen to be transported from the lungs to the muscles

- Acceleration of the heart rate five-fold to move greater quantities of blood, and thus, energy to the larger muscles

- Tensing of the muscles to prepare for "springing" action

- Release of chemicals into the blood that will make it clot faster should there be an injury

- Breakdown of body proteins to create glucose, which instantly fuels the muscles for greater energy

- Increase in perspiration to help cool the body

All of these changes are brought about by the elevation of three hormones: norepinephrine, epinephrine (more commonly known as adrenaline), and cortisol. Their release is critical to our survival in emergency situations. However, in a non-emergency situation, where their presence is unwarranted, they can actually be toxic.

Although the possibility of having to confront a wild tiger today is highly unlikely, we all have this response programmed deep within our unconscious mind. Moreover, while today's "tigers" don't sport stripes and saber-teeth, they do elicit the same stress response in many of us. Today's tigers are the stressors we discussed earlier such as rush-hour traffic. To a greater or lesser degree, these rather common events elicit the same primitive physiological response in our body. Although they are not life-threatening, the human tendency is to react as though they were. In addition, there are some individuals who do not necessarily need a particular event to instigate this response, but live in a chronic state of elevated arousal, with tense muscles, elevated heart rate, stomach churning, chronic headaches, backaches, insomnia, sweaty palms, and anxiety.

Earlier I mentioned that an estimated 75 percent of doctor visits are for stress-related illness. You may be asking yourself how feelings of stress can determine whether or not you get sick. To better understand this relationship, it is necessary to examine the human immune system.

STRESS AND THE IMMUNE SYSTEM

The immune system is fascinating and highly complex. It functions as a police force, whose job is to patrol the body in search of "non-self" invaders. These invaders, commonly referred to as antigens, may include (but are not limited to) bacteria, viruses, and parasites. As we have recently learned, an antigen does not have to be a germ or bacteria – artificial breast implants are detected by the body as "non-self" and cause immune responses in many women who have them.

The immune system is made up of a variety of highly specialized cells, each with a specific job to perform in the process of defending the body. The most common are the white blood cells. One type of white blood cell, the T-cell, helps in identifying foreign matter. Other white blood cells known as macrophages are programmed to recognize and ingest all antigens as well as cellular debris. Macrophages also "present" antigens to the T-cells. Natural killer, or NK cells, are responsible for acting against tumor and virus-affected cells.

Research has demonstrated that the hormones released during a stress response (particularly cortisol) have the effect of suppressing the immune system by reducing the number of T-cells. The most recent discoveries in mind-body research have revealed an extremely complex network of chemical messengers known as neuropeptides. Once regarded simply as hormones, further research has revealed these communication molecules to be more sophisticated than the classic hormone or neurotransmitter. More important, these neuropeptides appear to have an even more powerful and direct effect on immune function than any of the hormones studied to date.

Research conducted by Candace Pert, director of brain biochemistry at the National Institute of Mental Health, confirms that the mind and the nervous, endocrine, and immune systems are linked and communicate by way of tiny molecules secreted not only by the brain and immune system, but by the nerve cells of many other organs. It has been discovered that receptors for neuropeptides are highly concentrated in the areas of the brain that mediate emotion, as well as on the cells of the immune system itself.

Through immunological studies, scientists have been able to witness how our mental state can specifically affect the function of these neuropeptides and, consequently, the functioning of the cells of the immune system. States of anxiety, fear, anger, and depression, when prolonged, can have a debilitating effect on immune function. "What we see," says Dr. Joan Borysenko, former director of the Mind/Body Clinic, Harvard Medical School, "is a rich and intricate two-way communication system linking the mind, the immune system, and potentially all other systems, a pathway through which our emotions — our hopes and fears — can affect the body's ability to defend itself." Deepak Chopra, M.D., author of *Ageless Body, Timeless Mind*, explains, "Since your immune cells and endocrine glands are outfitted with the same receptors for brain signals as your neurons, they are like an extended brain."

So, together with hormones, the brain, and the immune system, neuropeptides and their receptors join in a communication network that, according to Candace Pert, represents the substrata of emotions.

Some of the most convincing scientific evidence of this thought-chemical interplay has come from the use of Positron Emission Tomography (PET) scans. PET scans can measure cerebral blood flow and volume as well as oxygen uptake, and have enabled researchers to watch the thinking process affect these measurements. Radioimmunoassay (RIA), another highly sensitive diagnostic tool, can detect hormonal concentration changes as an individual's thoughts and appraisals of a situation change.

IT'S NOT BUGS, BUT WHAT'S BUGGING YOU

Both the onset and duration of many illnesses may be dramatically influenced by our thoughts and feelings. Until recently, it was standard to attribute the onset of an illness to some unseen "bug" or virus. Yet we now know that pathogens (germs, bacteria, and viruses) are everywhere, and that each of us is constantly being exposed to them. In fact, many of these microbes quietly live within our bodies as dormant residents. For example, it has been found that some individuals can carry the cholera bacteria in their body yet not develop the disease. Similarly, far more people carry the HIV virus than have developed full-blown AIDS. What we are learning is that illness may be much less the result of the presence of a pathogen than it is one's vulnerability to that presence. The degree to which people are vulnerable to disease has much to do with the way they respond to their environment and the events in their lives. Each of us has a choice about how we respond to events; some responses are more conducive to health while others leave us more vulnerable. A stress response can elicit changes in our nervous system and hormone levels that will ultimately compromise the functioning of our immune system.

Volumes of studies exist on how specific events in people's lives can cause a measurable depression in the function of the immune system. Students are exceptionally qualified candidates for the study of stress and its effects, particularly when they are nearing an exam. In one study it was found that students' T-cell response to antigens was decreased beginning six weeks prior to an exam and lasting as long as two weeks afterward. In another study, medical students approaching exam time showed a decrease of interlukin-2, another chemical component of the immune system. Interlukin-2 is critical in defending the body against cancer.[109]

Sleep deprivation is another type of stress that depresses immune function. In one study where subjects were deprived of sleep for between 48 and 77 hours, there was a marked reduction in the response of phagocytes, immune cells that normally engulf and "digest" foreign bacteria and viruses.

It has been found that chronic grieving, a more passive form of emotional stress often brought about by the loss of a loved one, can cause the same biochemical imbalance as the constant elicitation of the fight or flight response. Consequently, this intense emotional suffering can have a dramatic effect on immune function. Most subjects who are grieving show a suppression of B-cells and T-cells, as well as a significant drop in the activity of NK cells. In one study conducted by researcher Anne O'Leary at Rutgers State University, a whopping 50 percent drop in NK cell activity was seen in bereaved individuals. NK cells are of particular significance, since they are responsible for destroying tumor cells.

An extremely depressed individual "projects sadness everywhere in [her] body – the brain's output of neurotransmitters becomes depleted, hormone levels drop, the sleep cycle is interrupted, neuropeptide receptors on the outer surface of skin cells become distorted, platelet cells in the blood become stickier and more prone to clump, and even [her] tears contain different chemical traces than tears of joy."[110] So powerful is the act of grieving that of the estimated

35,000 deaths occurring annually among the recently widowed in the United States, 7,000 may be directly linked to the death of a spouse.

STRESS AND HEART DISEASE

The repercussions of chronic stress are not limited to suppression of the immune system. Another major concern is the development of heart disease.

In the chapter "Diseases and Diet" in Book One, we looked at coronary heart disease as a consequence of a diet rich in fats and cholesterol. However, heart disease, and the atherosclerotic process that causes it, are not only affected by diet. The stress response can also influence this disease by causing platelet clumping, artery spasms, and injury to the arterial wall.

As mentioned earlier, one of the effects of the stress response brought about by the release of norepinephrine and epinephrine is that the blood platelets will clump together more easily in order to stem bleeding in the event of an injury. Interestingly, after blood platelets begin to clump together, they begin releasing another biochemical called thromboxane A2, which actually further stimulates platelets to stick together. This is helpful and necessary, if you have sustained an injury, to prevent excessive bleeding. However, without an injury, these sticky platelets continue to flow through the blood and become a risk factor.

As you now know, during the stress response, blood pressure is temporarily elevated by the constriction of the blood vessels and accelerated heart rate. By definition, blood pressure is a measurement of the force being exerted against the walls of the blood vessels. When the heart contracts and pushes blood into the arteries, the pressure is systolic. When the heart relaxes, the pressure is reduced (known as diastolic pressure). The higher a blood pressure reading, the greater the force is against the walls.

By design, the blood vessel network in the body is composed of larger vessels branching to progressively smaller and smaller vessels, a process known as bifurcation. This network begins with the largest vessel, known as the aorta, and continues branching into progressively smaller vessels until it reaches the smallest, the arterioles.

The intersection where a large vessel branches into two smaller ones is particularly vulnerable to wear by the turbulence generated by the constricted arteries. The greater the pressure, the more impact the flow can have at these branching points. As the walls are taxed for longer periods of time, the normally smooth lining of the vessel wall may develop small tears. An injury site like this is like a magnet to sticky platelets. As they float past the point of injury, they can become lodged in the torn tissue. Eventually, the injury site begins to accumulate a thick layer of platelets and other debris, and plaque forms. As the plaque increases, the diameter of the blood vessel becomes narrowed, thereby preventing blood flow and, thus, oxygen to the most important muscle of the body, the heart. When such deprivation occurs in coronary arteries, the result can be a heart attack; in the carotid artery, the result is a stroke.

An important study supporting this phenomenon was conducted by researchers at the University of Western Ohio. Volunteers in the study were asked to participate in a diabolical computer game, in which they had to identify the color that names of colors were printed in. For example, the word "blue" might have appeared on the screen in the color red. As the rate at which the words appeared increased, the volunteers became increasingly frustrated, and, consequently, their blood pressure levels rose.

The importance of the study became apparent during the two-year follow-up period. During this time, the volunteers' carotid arteries (the arteries leading to the brain) were examined for obstruction, using magnetic resonance imagery (MRI). The researchers discovered that those volunteers who responded to the test with the greatest degree of frustration and experienced the greatest increases in blood pressure also had developed the most significant arterial plaque.

Another possible outcome from stress is an arterial spasm. The lining of the arteries is composed of smooth muscle tissue. Like any other muscle in the body, this tissue can spasm. An arterial spasm results in the shutting down of normal blood flow in an artery.

Each of the above factors presented is a significant risk on its own. However, consider the combination of the three and you see how easily a heart attack or stroke can occur. These processes don't even take into account the possibility that arteries already have some plaque accumulation as the result of a poor diet, which only compounds the risk.

Clearly, we can see that our emotional state can significantly impact our overall health. Fortunately, there is much we can do to maintain emotional homeostasis. In the following chapters we will examine specific strategies for identifying specific triggers that may lead to elevated emotional states that can be a threat to our health. We will also look at specific tools we can use both to diffuse volatile emotional states as well as those that can be used as a form of "emotional maintenance."

CHAPTER TWENTY-SIX

STRESS MANAGEMENT

Most of the time you can't fight and you can't flee, but you can learn to flow.
– Robert S. Eliot

We will never be able to eliminate stressful events from our life entirely. However, we can control the degree to which we experience stress in our daily life and thus reduce the chances of compromising our well-being.

Stress management is about conditioning the mind and body so that a stress reaction is less likely to happen at all, and if it does, an individual has some means of diffusing an inappropriate response before it takes a serious toll on the body. We know that our perception of events and our response to them determine the degree to which we experience stress. While an event may carry stress potential, it is our interpretation that determines its power.

One of the first things we must do to reduce the amount of stress we experience is to learn to recognize *when* we are experiencing stress. We must also learn which events in our lives trigger that feeling and how we respond to those events. Most of us unconsciously react to stressors in a pattern established through repetition – one that is often disabling. We can learn, instead, to *consciously respond* to the same events in a way that will be empowering. Once we can recognize stress, we can utilize coping strategies. Further, we can inoculate ourselves to be more resistant to stress by practicing exercises, such as deep relaxation, visualization, and meditation, at times when we are in relatively non-stressful states.

into the next step. Immediately, you state a *belief* about this event or driver in the form of self-talk. While we have the choice of many beliefs, some of us fall into the trap of choosing an irrational one, such as the driver intentionally cut us off. Your self-talk might go something like this: "He saw me; he knew I was there; he intentionally did that" or "That maniac nearly killed me." This negative interpretation of the event is now going to elicit the stress response. Your perception is that you have lost control; you are being threatened. Now you move to the third step, *consequence*. Because your belief is negative and/or irrational, your actions will likely be negative as well. You might suddenly push the accelerator to the floor and take off in hot pursuit of this "maniac" who "nearly killed me." If you do, what do you think will be happening to your body? By this point, a flood of stress hormones has been released – you have chosen to fight. Your heart begins racing, blood pressure rises, muscles tense, fingers grip the steering wheel tightly, your breath is rapid and shallow, and even worse, nothing, not another car or person, seems to matter more than apprehending your offender. This is a clear example of the fight aspect of the "fight or flight" response.

Apply this same process to any situation; for example, being called in for a conference with your boss. You move through the same ABC process. The problem arises if in stage B you choose to fall back on an irrational or negative belief about a situation. Imagine that you have just received a less-than-friendly look from your employer (*activating event*). Your self-talk kicks in and you say something like, "Oh, no, he is mad at me, unhappy with my performance" (*belief*). This is a negative belief that may lead to irrational thoughts, followed by anxiety and physical stress. Perhaps, in an effort to avoid these thoughts, you take flight and suddenly leave the office (*consequence*).

What might be a more positive or rational response to this event? In order to move toward such a response, examine the empirical evidence surrounding a given situation. For instance, you may consider the fact that you had recently received accolades for your outstanding performance in the office. You may also consider that if your boss was ever concerned about something in the past, he addressed the issue directly with you. This objective information will support you in maintaining a more reasonable response. Rational self-talk might be, "The boss doesn't look very happy; maybe he had a bad night, didn't get enough sleep, or received some bad news." You can assemble your empirical evidence simply by doing what we call a "reality check." This simply involves asking yourself a few questions such as, "How has my performance been?" "Is there something I've done that would put me in a negative light with the boss?" Chances are that when you ask these questions, you'll get some clear answers that will quickly diffuse any negative beliefs.

Another great example is incorrect assumptions in personal relationships, such as when a person decides that someone she knows doesn't like her. When she's around him, she constantly feels uncomfortable because she "knows" he doesn't like her. When asked how she knows he doesn't like her, she has no rational answer. When she performs a "reality check," she can find no evidence to support her belief. "Did he say he doesn't like you?" "Has he ever offended you?" "Have you ever even talked to this man?" "If all your answers are 'no,' how do you know he doesn't like you?" "Because whenever I come near him in the office, he looks away." On a rational level, we all know that someone turning away could mean anything. In this woman's case, it meant nothing negative; in fact, it was just the opposite. It turned out that the man who was avoiding her was so infatuated with her he couldn't even look directly at her without becoming flustered.

I know a man who, whenever he flies on airplanes and hears an unusual noise, believes the plane is going to crash. His self-talk is, "This plane will crash. This is it; it's an old plane," and his mind is filled with images of planes crashing into the ground in a ball of flames. By the time the plane lands, he is physically taxed, having sat with muscles tensed, knuckles white, teeth gritted, and perspiring for the entire flight. His belief is totally irrational as it has no basis in fact or past experience. Positive self-talk could have quickly changed his emotional state and thus his physiological state, protecting him from an unhealthy stress response.

Let's review the steps we can take in preventing and diffusing irrational self-talk and the stress that can follow.

IDENTIFY IRRATIONAL OR NEGATIVE BELIEFS

The first step one must take is to identify irrational beliefs or negative self-talk: stage two of the ABC sequence. After an activating event, we must stop and examine what we have allowed to become emotional habit.

A helpful approach to identifying negative self-talk is to be on the lookout for expressions like "I have to," "I must," and "I should," and words like "horrible," "terrible," and "impossible." Watch for self-degrading remarks like "I'm stupid," "I really screwed up," "I'll never get it right," or "I can't." Keep in mind that thoughts are elusive. They not only occur in a quick, reflexive manner, but are often presented in an abbreviated fashion. For example, though in our minds we may only hear "stupid" or "gonna flunk," we need to expand these to a sentence ("I am stupid" or "I am going to flunk"). Examine these ideas carefully to determine the entire thought. Once we have effectively identified our irrational beliefs, we can move to the second step, refuting irrational beliefs.

REFUTING IRRATIONAL BELIEFS

Refuting irrational beliefs can be done by asking yourself some simple questions. Consider the medical student who is experiencing anxiety about an upcoming exam. Her irrational belief may be, "I'm going to flunk this exam; I just know it."

In order to refute this belief (and any other irrational belief), three questions should be asked:

1. *What evidence is there to support this belief?*

2. *What evidence is there that would prove this belief to be false?*

3. *What is the worst possible outcome of this situation?*

As you address these questions, write down your answers on a piece of paper. Write down any *rational* evidence that might support your idea. During this process you'll often find that there is little evidence to support the original belief. It can be very enlightening (and often astonishing) to discover that your beliefs have little substance. If you are honest with yourself and accept only rational evidence, you will likely find that these three questions take much of the wind out of your sails. Not only do you find no evidence for an irrational, negative belief, but there is often an abundance of evidence to support a positive one.

Finally, it is important to ask what the worst possible outcome of the situation might be. Too often we allow ourselves to become overwhelmed by situations that have little significance in the big picture. A helpful way to think about this is to look at how frames are used with art. Depending on the color, texture, and width, a frame can have varying effects on the art it contains. Have you ever taken a picture or photograph to a frame store and tried some of the sample frames? This can be fun. Doing so shows you how important the frame can be in presenting a piece of art. Some quiet and subtle artwork can be brought to life and given power simply by placing it in a dramatic frame. Complex and detailed work, conversely, can actually be muted with a more subtle frame. We can choose to frame a situation with thin, plain frames of little color or grandiose, ornately carved, gold-painted distractions that outweigh the work that they surround.

The reality is, more often than not, we frame our life experiences with inappropriate frames. We take little, insignificant works and surround them with flashy, loud, ornate borders that demand too much attention. As Dr. Robert Eliot says, "Rule No. 1 is, don't sweat the small stuff; rule No. 2 is, it's all small stuff." If you think about it, most of our problems are simply minor setbacks or inconveniences, yet we frame them as life-altering catastrophes.

Once you have identified your irrational thoughts, tested them with the questions above, and gained a more accurate perspective of the issue at hand, you can begin to replace your irrational self-talk with rational self-talk. Here are some examples:

Irrational self-talk:

This situation is hopeless; it'll never get any better for me.

Rational replacement self-talk:

No situation is hopeless; there is always something
I can do to influence my situation.

Irrational self-talk:

The boss is mad at me; my days are numbered at work.

Rational replacement self-talk:

The boss may be unhappy with himself.
I'll ask him/her if there is a problem.

Irrational self-talk:

I have to do this.

Rational replacement self-talk:

I don't have to do anything; I choose to do this because
of the advantage it offers me.

Irrational self-talk:

I'm no good at this; I'll never do it well.

Rational replacement self-talk:

I am only as skilled as I practice to be.
What can I do to increase my level of skill?

Irrational self-talk:

This plane is making a strange noise; I think it's going to crash.

Rational replacement self-talk:

I know that this is just one of thousands of flights around
the world that takes off everyday and lands safely.

or

The mechanics who work on these planes are experts who
know that our lives are in their hands.

or

Flying is much safer than driving a car. In fact, I'm in about
the safest place I could be for the next two hours.

You now have an effective way of disarming the irrational and unhealthy thoughts that may run through your mind and lead to states of stress. Now that you are conscious of the process, you can quickly begin your "thought patrol," looking as a detective does for damaging thoughts to refute. Then you can replace those thoughts with rational self-talk. While rational replacement self-talk is important and effective in disarming irrational thinking, it is important that you apply the second step and ask, "What are my beliefs?"

Without asking yourself questions, it is easy sometimes to slip back into irrational or destructive thinking. However, most people find that if they ask the three questions and write the answers down, they will have permanently diffused misleading or negative thoughts and will be less likely to experience them again. Remember, it is through repetition that many of your irrational thoughts have come to be, and it will be through the same repetition that you will dissolve them forever.

ANTICIPATE CHALLENGING SITUATIONS

Much of the stress we experience in life comes from feeling out of control. One way to help ourselves retain a sense of control is to anticipate challenging situations that may act as stressors. Some situations arise with no warning at all, yet we are exposed to others with greater frequency.

Commute traffic, which I mentioned earlier, is always a good example, as many of us contend with it daily. Despite this, many of us also respond to it with great agitation as though it were something unusual. Becoming emotional about the situation will have no bearing on the traffic problem. The freeway won't suddenly unclog itself. The healthier approach is to view the situation in advance and choose to use it as an opportunity. In this case, ask yourself what you can do with the time. For some, turning on classical music is very relaxing. For others, listening to self-improvement tapes or audio books is a positive, life-enhancing solution. You can use a small cassette recorder to take "verbal notes" of things you need to do or people to contact. Later, you can transfer these notes to a legal pad or Day Runner™. Another option these days is the use of a hands-free cellular phone. Perhaps you can make needed calls during the commute home and save yourself time later. Any one of these options is a way of influencing your situation. No longer are you the "victim" of commute traffic, a feeling that can lead to frustration, anxiety, and the physiological changes we looked at earlier. You can think of your car as a "rolling classroom" where an "educational course" can start in a moment's notice.

When I am on an airplane that has suddenly been delayed on the runway, it always amazes me that as soon as the captain announces the delay, there is usually a group of people who gasp loudly, throw their hands up in the air, and then engage in chit chat with comrades over how frustrating and unfair the situation has become. Some become angry, even abusive. Yet when I look around, I always notice a few individuals who appear not to have heard the announcement. They get out their personal cassette players, open up a good book, or simply get to know the person seated next to them. These people know better than to allow a situation that is out of their control to get to them. Instead, they use the temporary setback as an opportunity.

Becoming stuck in traffic on the freeway or on a runway are very real possibilities for many of us. So it is important that we anticipate such events in advance and be prepared to utilize the time in a constructive manner that keeps us "in control." As a rule, always carry a laptop computer, book, cassette tapes, or other materials that you can refer to in times when you are temporarily "on hold" in lines or in traffic.

CHAPTER TWENTY-SEVEN

TIME MANAGEMENT

Failing to plan is planning to fail.
– Anonymous

Another important step in preventing stressful feelings is the effective planning of our time. Without such planning, we are more liable to make inappropriate decisions that eat up important time and lead to frustration, anxiety, and stress. Without effective time management, we are likely to end up rushing to events and appointments, feeling overwhelmed, and lacking "down time" for relaxation.

MAKE A "TO DO" LIST

If you don't already do so, use a weekly planner or notepad to write down appointments, activities, and other commitments. This simple process is very effective for relieving feelings of anxiety and stress.

I always carry a legal pad with two to three pages of things that need to be done. I call it my "paper brain." Throughout the day I cross things off as I complete them and add new things as they come to mind. It's much easier to remain level-headed when I know I have a schedule. People without lists tend to have difficulty relaxing because they are always wondering what they should be doing or if they have forgotten something. They often end up preoccupied with daily trivialities without a list to remind them of vital concerns. Those without lists are usually frustrated by their lack of progress, wondering at the end of the day why they failed to accomplish more. This group is also much more likely to suffer insomnia. In contrast, people with clearly defined schedules are less likely to suddenly fly out the door or race through traffic to make a forgotten appointment. At the end of the day, they can look at their lists and see the items that have been crossed off, giving them tremendous feelings of accomplishment and a sense that they are in control of the direction of their lives.

Start your list today, writing down everything you plan to accomplish tomorrow. Don't fill your list with insignificant time killers. Only write down key items – things that have true importance in your life and that will propel you forward. It's easy to come up with a list of things to keep yourself busy. Yet being busy does not necessarily mean being productive. One can easily spend a whole day doing much but achieving little. Chinese philosopher Lin Yutang put it eloquently when he said, "Besides the noble art of getting things done, there is the noble art of leaving things undone. The wisdom in life consists in the elimination of non-essentials."

When making the list, place items in order of importance. The most important items should be at the top of your list and receive first priority. In prioritizing your items, a good question to ask yourself is, "If I only had time to do one item on this list tomorrow, which would I do?" Your answer should go to the top of the list. Then ask yourself what you would do if you could squeeze another item in, and continue formulating your list in this manner. At the end of each day, look at your list and place any leftover items on the top of your list for the next day. Make your weekly list on Sunday evenings and make your daily list each night before you go to bed. If you have never used lists before, I guarantee you will be surprised by the increase in your level of productivity in a short period.

TAKE ACTION AT ONCE

How often have you rediscovered something, such as a letter or memo you need to respond to, a term paper assignment, or other responsibility, and wished that you had taken care of it immediately? We are all guilty of procrastination at some level, and usually it comes back to haunt us when we have other priorities to attend to.

To prevent a sudden cascade of "leftovers" at the end of the week or month, take action on simple items immediately. When faxes, letters, and phone calls come in, if you can respond to them immediately, do so.

CHAPTER TWENTY-EIGHT

GOAL SETTING

A life without goals is like a ship without a rudder.
Anonymous

If you are reading this book in its entirety before beginning the exercise routines provided, pay special attention to this section. In fact, have a pen and some paper handy to jot down important notes.

There is a saying that goes, "If you don't know where you are going, you'll probably end up somewhere else." I would add that you'll probably end up there in a highly stressed and dissatisfied state. Many people have no clear idea where they are headed. They assume little control over the direction of their lives and, as a result, end up being victims of fate.

I believe that goal setting is probably the single most powerful tool we have at our disposal. Ironically, few people use it. In fact, the majority of folks will spend more time plotting out their next vacation, Christmas wish list, or weekly grocery list than they will ever spend establishing a list of lifetime goals. Statistics indicate that only about 5 percent of the population have established goals for themselves.

When we don't have clearly defined goals, we are more prone to stress because our approach to life has less planning and structure. Consequently, we become more like a passenger in the runaway car of fate rather than a driver in control of the direction we are heading. Ultimately, our level of productivity in all areas of our life becomes severely compromised and that invaluable commodity called time slips by, barely used to our advantage.

The reason goal setting is so powerful is that, by nature, we are goal-seeking animals. In fact, in our subconscious minds we have a cybernetic quality that might be thought of as a goal-seeking mechanism. Like a heat-seeking missile, this mechanism is extremely effective once it has a clearly defined target.

I look at goal-setting as being part of a blueprint drawing process. If you told a contractor that you wanted to build a house, the first thing he would ask for would be the blueprints. Without them, he would have no clear picture of what type of home you have in mind. The same goes for any endeavor including exercising your body. To a degree, you are the architect of your body. Before you start a program, you need to outline what you wish to achieve. What are you interested in? Building? Sculpting? Shaping? Reducing? To what degree? Most people take what they get, but what they get can rarely be considered success. Others have ideas or wishes, but until they are clearly defined and written down, these are not goals on which they can focus. Goal setting is important because it lifts us out of mediocrity. When you set goals, you push yourself out of the "comfort zone" and into the "achievement zone." This applies to other aspects of your life as well, including your career or business, education, relationships, and family life.

An important study showing the power of goal setting was conducted with the Yale graduates of the class of 1953. At that time, the graduates were interviewed to see how many had established clearly defined goals. It turned out that only 3 percent had established goals for themselves. Then in 1973, these same graduates were interviewed again. It was found that those 3 percent who had established clearly defined goals for themselves had achieved more than the entire 97 percent who had failed to define their goals.

We need to have clear goals regarding all areas of our lives:

• family and friends (relationship with spouse, children, friends) • career (advancement, certifications and licensing, employer-employee relationships) • education (self-education, language courses, seminars, books, tapes) • finances (budgeting expenses, savings, investments) • community (volunteer work, local government, environmental issues) • self-improvement • health and fitness. These are some of the most important goals to examine.

Take some time to consider each of these areas and the goals you have in each. What do these goals mean to you? What will they bring to your life and the lives of others? Write your ideas down on paper. Some people effectively determine what their goals are but fail to write them down. Writing down your goals is another way of "programming" the mind. It's also an important step toward commitment. Without committing your goals to paper they remain only wishes.

Be very specific in writing down your goals. "I want to get in better shape" is too vague and leaves no specifics on which you can focus. "I want to have a 31-inch waist" or "I intend to have 18-inch biceps" is specific. "I plan to be free of hypertension medication" is another specific goal. These goals are your long-term goals, and although they might even seem impossible to attain at first, if they are reduced to smaller, incremental goals, the picture changes significantly.

I once coached a man who was primarily interested in achieving great strength from his training. His goal was to make dramatic increases in the poundages he could lift. Specifically, he wanted to be able to perform the squat exercise with 315 pounds of weight – an ambitious goal. At the time we met, he was performing squats with 165 pounds. You may consider the difference, an increase of 150 pounds, overwhelming. However, what we did together is break the long-term goal of 315 down to a series of short-term goals. I explained that if he were to aim for a 15-pound increase per month, which is quite reasonable when considering the rate at which the thigh muscles increase in strength, 10 months later he would be squatting 315 pounds. Each month there was the "mini-reward" of reaching the next short-term goal, and that served to inspire him to move on to the next level.

This same process applies to any goal you have. The key is in breaking down the larger goal into manageable chunks. Perhaps your goal in education is to earn an advanced degree. While the degree is your long-term major goal, you will need to break it down into manageable smaller goals such as preparing to take a college entrance exam or enrolling in an exam preparatory course.

Perhaps you wish to lose some weight. First, you must establish a long-term goal. For example, let's say that your long-term goal is to permanently lose 25 pounds of body weight. By incorporating regular exercise and the Revised American Diet, this is a goal you certainly can achieve and maintain! However, you must break that goal down into smaller short-term goals. Let's say your short-term goal will be to lose two pounds of body weight a week, a very safe and manageable goal. By making a commitment to lose two pounds a week, you can effectively achieve your long-term goal in 12 weeks.

As I mentioned earlier, the reason goal setting is so effective is that our minds have a cybernetic quality. Like an "auto-pilot" system, this goal-seeking mechanism works very effectively once it has a course to follow.

Here are some hints for successful goal achievement:

1. Make your goal realistic and incremental. Don't "overshoot" and demand too much in too short a time period.

2. Write your goal down. Then rewrite your goal regularly at the beginning of each week. By rewriting your goal you will be deeply programming your mind and helping keep priorities on the "surface." Writing your goal early in the morning is a good way to keep it at the top of your mental priority list and will sensitize you to information and circumstances throughout the day that may enable you to move toward your goal more quickly.

3. Be specific and detailed in writing your goal. If you want a promotion, to what position do you desire to be promoted? How do you wish to be compensated?

4. Use a calendar and indicate specific dates by which you plan to achieve your goal. Without deadlines, you have no way of quantifying your progress.

5. Set short-term goals (from weeks to months), long-term goals (from months to years), and lifetime goals.

6. Update your goals regularly. With time you will reach certain goals; others may change and need to be refined or expanded.

7. Use the art of visualization to see yourself already having achieved your goal.

CHAPTER TWENTY-NINE

LEARNING TO RELAX

Nothing can bring you peace but yourself.
– Ralph Waldo Emerson

Since a state of relaxation is the antithesis of a state of physical stress, it is clear how important relaxation exercises can be, both during times of stress and when we are more relaxed, as a means of further inoculating ourselves against a stressful reaction in the first place. The more we practice relaxation exercises, the less likely that muscular tension and stress will accumulate within our body.

Janice Kiecolt-Glaser, a research psychologist at Ohio State University, has demonstrated that not only are those who practice relaxation skills less likely to become stressed, but they will also show improved immune function. In one study, medical students were found to have a lowered T-cell count on the day of examinations. After the students were taught relaxation exercises, their T-cell count increased, according to how much they practiced. In other words, the more they practiced relaxation skills, the stronger their immune system became.

BREATHING

In the exercise section, we looked at the importance of proper breathing while exercising. Deep breathing is an instant antidote to feelings of stress. It releases feelings of tension in the muscles and has a wonderful calming effect on the emotions.

Even during a moderately stressful response, our breathing is likely to become quick and shallow. In full-blown stress reactions, our breathing may become excessively rapid and shallow. This is called hyperventilation. Few of us think about our breath throughout the day. Even when we are not exposed to a stressor, our breathing is likely to be shallow. Shallow breathing expels less carbon dioxide from the lungs and takes in less life-supporting oxygen to the lungs and the rest of the body. When we breathe deeply, we can bring in up to seven times more oxygen than with unconsciously shallow breathing.

ABDOMINAL BREATHING

Most of us are chest-breathers. When we breathe with our chest, our abdomen moves in when we inhale and out when we exhale. However, abdominal breathing allows us to utilize the full capacity of our lungs. In abdominal breathing, the abdomen expands as we inhale and pulls in as we exhale. This type of breathing results in more room for the lungs to expand and contract, and, thus, more fresh oxygen intake and more carbon dioxide release.

Take a moment right now to learn the difference between abdominal and chest breathing. Sit up straight in a chair or on the edge of a bed. Place one hand on your abdomen area. Slowly inhale deeply, allowing your abdominal muscles to expand. Then exhale fully, pulling the abdominal muscles in tightly. You will notice that the tighter you pull in your abdominal muscles, the more air will be forced out of your lungs. Take another couple of deep breaths and practice making your abdominal muscles expand outward on the inhalation and contract inward on the exhalation.

Deep abdominal breathing is something you can practice each day. Begin your mornings with two or three minutes of deep abdominal breathing. You will feel refreshed and energized. At times when you feel yourself becoming stressed, you can quickly diffuse the feelings and return to a state of deep calm simply by performing several deep abdominal breaths in succession.

Not only is relaxation an effective means for diffusing feelings of anxiety and tension, numerous studies have demonstrated that, after periods of relaxation, levels of the stress hormones (cortisol, adrenaline) that can impair immune function drop significantly.[112] Studies have also shown that after periods of deep relaxation, T-cell counts that were previously depressed through high stress became elevated to more normal levels. The more one relaxes, the more one's T-cell count rises.

Relaxation is something we can use both when we are in a stressful situation, and something we can practice regularly as a form of maintenance.

Some people believe that they are very relaxed throughout the day. Yet even those who work in the most hassle-free, low-stress environments experience physical and emotional stresses they are not aware of. You may or may not be very relaxed at this moment as you read these words. Check your shoulders. Are they tight and retracted? Try letting your shoulders drop, releasing them as though they were very heavy. Were you previously holding them tightly? Now check your jaw. Is it clenched? Are you grinding your teeth? Allow your jaw to become heavy, release it and let it drop. Are your toes clenched in your shoes? Many of us hold parts of our body in tight and clenched positions, even in relaxed situations. Doing this uses energy. Yet we have been doing it so long that we are not even aware of it. After using the following relaxation techniques, you will become much more aware of the subtle ways in which we create physical tension. With practice, you will be able to bring your body easily into a deeply relaxed state, regardless of the activity or situation.

THE TENSION-RELEASE METHOD

The Tension-Release Method is one effective way to relax. By experiencing your muscles in a high state of tension, you will better be able to recognize when your muscles "slip" into such a state. By tensing and then relaxing your muscles, you will enable them to relax much more deeply than by simply trying to relax mentally. This exercise involves moving through the entire musculature of the body, tensing and then relaxing small groups of muscles, one at a time.

Choose a time when you will be free from interruption. Lie down on a bed or the floor and close your eyes. Begin by taking four deep breaths. Inhale deeply through your nose and exhale completely through your mouth. Place your arms at your sides, with your palms facing up and legs extended fully. You will progressively tense every muscle in your body, either one at a time or in pairs.

You may prefer to begin at your head and work down to your feet or the reverse. It makes no difference. For example, begin at the head by raising your eyebrows as high as possible, and furrowing your forehead. Hold this tensed position for five seconds and then let go. Feel the muscles of your upper face relaxing. Move to your nose and eyes. Close both eye lids tightly while wrinkling your nose, hold them for five seconds, then release them. Moving to your mouth, make a broad and exaggerated smile, holding it for five seconds and releasing. Feel your face relaxing more deeply. Now move to your neck. Slowly pull your head up and bring your chin toward your chest, hold for five seconds, and relax. Now move your head backwards, feeling your neck crease. Hold and relax. Now raise your shoulders up toward your ears, tensing them for five seconds, and releasing. Moving to your upper arms, lock your elbows and tighten the tricep muscles of the back of your arms for five seconds and release them. Then curl your lower arm up and squeeze the bicep muscles tightly for five seconds and release. Now make a fist with each hand and squeeze the fists tightly for five seconds and release. Move to your stomach area and tighten your abdominal muscles for five seconds and release. Moving to your upper legs, lock your knees to tightly tense your thigh muscles for five seconds. To tense the lower leg muscles, aim your toes up toward you, with your heel out. Then push your toes away, pulling your heel in. Hold both of these positions for five seconds and relax them.

In one final contraction, squeeze all of the muscles you have covered simultaneously for five seconds, and then release them. Your body should feel thoroughly relaxed at this point. A very helpful addition is to softly instruct yourself with a "relax" each time you release a muscle that has been tensed. This will not only aid in your relaxation session, but you will begin to anchor the word relax with the feeling of a fully relaxed muscle. Then, in anxiety-provoking situations, you can simply scan your body to find areas that are tense and tell yourself to relax. This is an effective tool for getting in touch with tension.

With practice, you will become very sensitized to what your muscles feel like when they are tense and what they should feel like in a relaxed state. At that point, you will no longer need to move through this entire tension-release process. Instead you will simply be able to command yourself to relax and feel the deeply relaxed state in your muscles and body. Throughout the day you can do this Tension-Release Method on specific areas that you notice becoming tense. Perhaps it's your shoulders when you are seated at your office desk or your hands gripping the steering wheel of your car. You can perform this relaxation technique as a way of overcoming mild insomnia and assuring deep sleep. You can also use it before taking an exam or making a public presentation, or before an important interview.

VISUALIZATION

Your imagination is your preview of life's coming attractions.
– Albert Einstein

Visualization is a process whereby we use the imagination coupled with the senses to create rich images in our mind's eye. When utilized to its fullest potential, no other tool can so powerfully influence our ability to relax, prepare us for challenging events, and help us achieve goals. Visualization is really a very simple process, yet with relentless repetition it becomes a very powerful, life-shaping tool.

VISUALIZATION AND RELAXATION

After you have performed the Tension-Release Method to facilitate relaxation, you can employ visualization to take you to an even deeper level of relaxation. You can also use visualization separately at times when you are not able to move through an entire relaxation exercise such as tension-release.

There are many different images that can be visualized for relaxation, such as gazing at a mountain lake, watching clouds moving across the sky, drifting on a small boat at sea, sitting on a mountaintop, or walking down a deserted beach. Use the scene(s) you find most relaxing.

The key to successful visualization is making the experience as real as possible. This requires that you employ as many of your senses – including touch, taste, smell, and hearing – as you can. As an example, let's look at the image of a mountain lake through the visualization process. Either lying down or seated comfortably in a chair, and at a time when you are not likely to be disturbed, close your eyes and begin by taking 8-10 deep breaths. If you already have a specific lake in mind, you can use that as a springboard for the exercise; otherwise, begin by imagining a quiet mountain lake scene. Perhaps you find yourself lying on a chaise lounge or on a towel on top of a bed of small polished pebbles or grains of sand. In your mind's eye, look around and take note of your surroundings. Are you alone? Look out at the clear lake water. Is it smooth as glass or is there a slight breeze producing a ripple effect across the water? If there is a breeze, feel it gently move across your arms and face. Is there a scent in the breeze, perhaps pine or sweet flowers? Inhale the fresh mountain air deeply into your lungs. If there are trees nearby, can you hear the wind gently moving through the needles of the pine trees? If you are close to the lake shore, perhaps you can see a small pattern of ripples nudging against the sand.

This should give you an idea of the detail you can bring into your visualization experience. The more sensations you include, the more realistic the experience will become.

Initially, you may find your visualization process is interrupted by unwanted thoughts. This is common even for those of us who have practiced visualization for some time. What is important is not to become frustrated and tense. Simply remain relaxed and gently brush the distracting thought away. With practice, you will find it easier to let go, depart fully into your "mental vacation," and remain clear of any distracting thoughts.

VISUALIZATION AND GOAL ACHIEVEMENT

I like to think of visualization as a form of map making. In a way, you are creating a map for your subconscious mind to follow. With this map, your mind will create a blueprint to move you in the direction of achieving your goals. Sound complex? Actually, it's not. Your unconscious mind has the ability to instruct your conscious mind to carry out those images you imagine repeatedly. Visualization, as a sophisticated form of mental rehearsal, is a way you can help enrich and expedite this process.

To understand why the process of visualization is successful, you should know a bit more about the mind. You may have heard already that the mind can be divided into three parts, the conscious, the subconscious, and the unconscious. The unconscious mind is handling all the processes of the autonomic system, such as breathing and the heartbeat. It's also where information about your self-image (what you think of yourself) is stored. Think about the last hour and all the things that went through your mind on a conscious level. Though many of the things we think about are mundane, we are also constantly checking in with ourselves. We are evaluating our past and present performances, and making predictions of those to come, all based on previously stored information. We may be thinking about school performance, social interactions, meetings with clients, our children or spouse, or the next workout at the gym.

We program ourselves much like a computer is programmed by a technician. While we are not actually loading and unloading diskettes or punching in commands, our self-talk, daydreams, and other experiences are retained in a gigantic memory bank. In fact, we don't have to think consciously about storing the information; that's handled by the subconscious mind, which is always listening and committing information to memory. Why? Because the subconscious uses this information to move us in the direction of our most dominant thoughts. You see, the subconscious operates under the assumption that what we think about most, we want. Unfortunately, this goal-seeking mechanism does not distinguish between "good" and "bad" goals. It simply zeroes in on the thoughts and images we harbor in our minds. You have already seen the problems that occur when we dwell on negative thoughts. It can also be a problem if we dwell on negative images. The subconscious is a bit like a homing device. The target is what you think about most. When the subconscious has a clear image of what it is you want (when your thoughts, images, and ideas are clear to you), it will begin moving you in the direction of that target more efficiently.

Ask people who have won an athletic competition about the mental images they held. They will tell you how they saw themselves winning, heard the applause, and felt the incomparable feeling of victory long before the competition ever began. That is because people are not successful at achieving their goals by mistake! A power lifter does not pull 500 pounds off the floor by accident; a sprinter does not just happen to end up across the finish line a second earlier than her opponent. They have very clear pictures of what they want to achieve and how they will look and feel when they have reached their goal. Almost all successful athletes use visualization and will attest to its value. Yet this powerful tool should not be limited to athletic pursuits. It can be applied to your career, family, and personal relationship goals just as effectively.

The success of visualization can be partly attributed to a little-known fact about the mind. The subconscious is incapable of detecting a difference between reality and fantasy. Clinical psychologists have confirmed that the nervous system is unable to detect the difference between an event that actually occurs and one that has been imagined vividly. This is because a sufficient number of the neurons stimulated during an actual experience are also stimulated during the visualization process. So, those events that you visualize begin to overlap the actual experience. Therefore, what you dream in your conscious mind is stored in your subconscious as having actually occurred. Not only is there a vivid visual record of the event, but there is often a neurological response to it. This is why visualization is such a powerful tool.

Therefore, if you see yourself winning something over and over again, by the time the competition comes around, it's old hat. You have done it already; you know what to expect and feel. If a dancer visualizes her dance routine for a performance, step by step, each move exactly the way she wants it to look, she will be programming her subconscious mind for that performance. If a gymnast visualizes his routine performed flawlessly with repetition, he will have had more perfect practices than the gymnast who does not visualize. A public speaker can practice her presentation continuously, visualizing both her ideal performance and the audience responding with tremendous enthusiasm to what she has said.

Dr. Richard Suinn of Colorado State University is a consultant to the United States National Olympic Ski Team. He guides the ski team through a visualization process that many of the skiers say is so real they experience not only the sensations of the cold air and the hard snowpack, but even the twitching of muscles that would be used in the actual performance. Our Olympic athletes are now regularly using what the formidable Russian athletes discovered and began using many years ago.

In addition to improving athletic performance, there are many other areas of life in which visualization will maximize performance. For instance, I once used visualization techniques to prepare for a job interview. I knew I was going up against the best of the best for a top company. The company's recruiters were looking for people who could be relaxed and easygoing, individuals who could comfortably interact with a variety of persons in high-stress situations. Rather than get all worked up about the interview and what might happen, I began to create a skit in my mind of exactly how I wanted the interview to go. I paid careful attention to how I would speak, breathe, and sit. I felt my body relaxed and at ease. I even visualized how my interviewer would behave, which put me in an even more receptive and outgoing state for the actual interview. In other words, I rehearsed in my mind! When I got there I was all smiles. Though it was the real thing, it felt like just another repetition of something I had already experienced.

Visualization is an excellent tool for tackling all sorts of changes we might like to make because our mind moves us toward our current dominant thoughts. The clearer the images are in our mind, the more efficiently they become our reality. We can use the power of visualization in any area of our lives in which we would like to influence the outcome.

Visualization techniques can be used to work toward better communication with loved ones. Numerous studies have demonstrated the effectiveness of visualization to assist individuals with healing from various types of illness, including catastrophic illnesses.

Let's look more closely at the process of visualization for achieving your fitness goals.

To effectively visualize, you must be in a relaxed state. The more relaxed you are, the better. Some people have no problem relaxing and can even drift into cat naps at will. For others it isn't as easy. If you are one of those who needs more assistance, you can use the progressive relaxation exercise discussed earlier as a way to prepare for effective visualization.

To visualize a fitness goal, keep your eyes closed, and while lying down, create a clear, three-dimensional image of your body; not the body you presently possess, but the one you want, the totally fit physique for which you are exercising. Look at this figure from all angles, closely examining every detail of your body. You will find it helpful to start either from your toes or your head and then work in the opposite direction, first the front, then the back. Make sure to get a good look at the shape and symmetry of your muscles. Look at how your face is defined and clearly see every detail of the new you. The image you create may suddenly vanish. This is not unusual. Work to bring it back as soon as you can and continue doing so until you can hold that image for at least a couple of minutes. Now you will have a blueprint for your future body, which you can look at any time you wish and which will assist you in reaching your ideal physique much more effectively.

Now, take that physique into the gym. That's right, mentally go to the place where you exercise each day. You may want to start with upper-body exercises such as the bench press. Imagine vividly that you are lying down and will begin bench pressing. See the plates on the ends of the barbell. Take note of the poundages. It can be set at whatever weight you like, as long as it's realistic. See the dumbbells, barbells, or machine you may be exercising with, and get the feeling of exercising.

To further enhance this process, incorporate some of your other senses. The more senses you involve, the more effective the visualization will be. Imagine the sounds of the environment, for example, your gym. Hear the clanking of the weights or the turning gears of the machines. Get the feeling of your muscles contracting against the resistance of free weights or machines. Notice the temperature of the air and even the quality of light in the room.

As I mentioned before, athletes can use visualization to "preview" athletic events. They can see themselves winning the event, feel the trophy or medal in their hands, and hear the audience applauding with approval.

If you have a great fear of public speaking, you can use visualization to rehearse with great detail the way you would like the event to go. In a situation that is likely to arouse the stress response, with visualization practice, you can create the situation in vivid detail, and see and hear things go exactly as you would like. The result is that when the actual event occurs, your mind and body will have been pre-programmed to perform with ease and confidence. For instance, you can move through the entire performance, reading your speech. As you do so, you can vividly see yourself looking up and making eye contact with the audience, feeling relaxed and at ease. You can practice responding to questions that might come from the audience and hear them applaud with approval at the completion of the presentation.

WHEN TO VISUALIZE

There are a few key times to use visualization. The most effective times are just before falling asleep at night and just after waking in the morning. At these times, our minds have the least "mental traffic," and programming the mind occurs with greater clarity and ease. Other times may be just prior to going to the gym to exercise or before an important job interview or meeting. In terms of your exercise goals, it's a good idea to visualize your workouts before you do them. Understand what muscle groups you will be training and what you want the workout, the sets, and the reps to be like. Get a full sensory picture and feeling of how you want the workout to go; then do it that way! You can visualize just before any situation – an interview, an exam, a date, an athletic event – for which you desire a positive outcome. However, the farther in advance you begin using visualization, the more effective you'll find it to be.

CHAPTER THIRTY-ONE

MEDITATION

Within you there is a stillness and a sanctuary
to which you can retreat at any time and be yourself.
– Hermann Hesse

Every day we are exposed to countless people, events, sounds, thoughts, sensations, feelings, memories, and images. Even though we may go home at the end of the day and be in an environment with fewer people, events, and congestion, many of us continue to maintain a significant amount of mental traffic right up to the moment we fall asleep. The information can flow like a tap, flooding our minds with too much clutter. We may think something like, "It's getting late, better get to sleep...did I lock the door?...dinner was good...what's on the agenda for tomorrow...wow, I forgot to write that paper...oh, that TV show is on, I don't want to miss that...where is that paper I was reading? Whose dog is that barking?...wish I had a dog."

Meditation is a path away from this bombardment of internal and external stimuli; it is a mental retreat to a place of peace and quiet where the mind becomes calm. Meditation takes us out of the past and the future and brings us into the present. It is calming, yet at the same time heightens our awareness. It develops skill in concentration and focus, which in turn assist us in problem solving and successfully reaching goals.

Up until the early seventies, meditation had been largely ignored as a means of enhancing one's health. Many people erroneously believed that meditation is only associated with religion, finding God, becoming a cultist, or "becoming one with the universe." Without question, many regular meditators mention some spiritual experiences, but meditation can be and is most commonly practiced independently of any religious affiliation, philosophy, or belief.

Those who meditate regularly have demonstrated the ability not only to alleviate stressful feelings and achieve a deep state of relaxation, but also to reduce their blood pressure, heart rate, rate of respiration, and oxygen consumption. Long-term meditators have also been found to have lower levels of the stress hormones cortisol and adrenaline. Some researchers say that, because of these changes, long-term meditators can effectively slow the rate at which they age.

A study published in the journal *Hypertension* and led by researcher Robert Sneider, M.D., showed that regular meditation can have the same blood-pressure-lowering effect as medications currently used by hypertensives.

Other studies are demonstrating that not only does regular meditation play an important role in reducing stress, but it may also be effective in reducing cholesterol levels, chronic pain, and sleep disturbances.[111] In one study, five participants reduced their serum cholesterol by between 4 and 9 percent, and three by as much as 35 percent.[112] In another study, compared to those who did not meditate regularly, meditators showed 80 percent fewer cases of heart disease and 50 percent fewer cases of cancer.[113] The landmark Lifestyle Heart Trial conducted by Dean Ornish, M.D., and associates, demonstrated for the first time that atherosclerosis can be reversed through comprehensive lifestyle changes. An essential component of the stress reduction portion of this program included regular meditation.[114]

Like other forms of deep relaxation, meditation brings the body into a state that allows it to return to homeostasis. In this state, all of the interrelated systems, the immune system in particular, can function at their optimal level.

Meditation is really about reaching a state of mindfulness. Jon Kabat-Zinn, Ph.D., founder of the Stress Reduction Clinic at the University of Massachusetts Medical Center, describes this state as "paying attention in a particular way: on purpose, in the present moment, and non-judgmentally. This kind of attention nurtures greater awareness, clarity, and acceptance of present-moment reality. It wakes us up to the fact that our lives unfold only in moments. If we are not fully present for many of those moments, we may not only miss what is most valuable in our lives, but also fail to realize the richness and the depth of our possibilities for growth and transformation." As we saw in the section "Understanding Feelings that Lead to Stress," many of us are living far from the present. We spend our time and energy in the past and the future, being guided by a barrage of irrational thoughts, many at an unconscious level. In meditation, we can climb out of this mental traffic — the dreams, worries, thoughts, and fantasies of everyday — and become a quiet observer in a place of "pure awareness."

With practice, the awareness of the thoughts, feelings, and sensations you gain through your meditation will spill over into times when you are not meditating. This increased awareness or presence will help prevent irrational thoughts and debilitating reactions to stressors you may encounter and allow you to experience more enjoyment each minute of each day.

HOW TO MEDITATE

To experience successful meditation sessions, there are a few guidelines that should be followed.

1. Meditate at least an hour after eating because digestion will prevent you from being totally alert.

2. Choose a place that is quiet and where you are unlikely to be disturbed by a phone ringing or other interruptions.

3. Find a comfortable position that you can maintain for at least 20 minutes. A traditional position involves sitting on your knees with your big toes touching and buttocks resting on your feet. For some, sitting cross-legged, either on the floor or on a cushion, is most comfortable. Others sit with their legs extended straight before them and their back supported, while others choose to lie down or sit in a straight-back chair. Whatever is most comfortable is right.

There are two popular ways to meditate, one that involves counting breaths, and the other repeating what is known as a mantra. Experiment with both to see which is most effective for you.

BREATH-COUNTING MEDITATION

In breath-counting meditation, you breathe through your nose at all times. After finding yourself in a comfortable position, take a deep breath using the abdominal breathing style discussed earlier. As you exhale, say to yourself, "one." With each exhalation repeat to yourself "one." An alternative is to continue counting with each exhalation until you reach "four" and then return to "one."

Some people prefer counting to "one" because it takes their focus off of reaching a goal, even if that goal is simply to reach four, and makes it easier for them to stay in the present moment.

MANTRA MEDITATION

In mantra (*man* means "to think" and *tra* means "to liberate") meditation, you will be repeating a name or syllable throughout the meditation session. Common mantras used in the Eastern tradition are om, which means "I am," *so-ham*, which means "I am he," and *sa-ham*, which means "I am she." Yet a mantra does not necessarily need to have meaning to anyone other than yourself. It can simply be a sound or two syllables of your own choosing. You can also choose words such as "calm" or "relaxed" as your mantra.

Once you have chosen a mantra, begin your session by chanting the mantra aloud. After about five minutes, you may find yourself feeling centered and you can then chant silently to yourself.

With either breath counting or mantra chanting, the key to your meditative session is to remain calm and relaxed and not judge what is happening. Slow and deepen your breath and remain completely passive. If your mind begins to drift, gently bring the focus back to your breath, observing your inhalation and exhalation. With practice, you will find it easier and easier to remain focused and free of intruding thoughts. However, even advanced meditators become distracted by thoughts, and consider the process of noticing the phenomenon, and returning to breath, simply part of the practice. Do not become concerned over whether or not you are meditating properly. There should be no judgment about your meditation – just experience the calm and relaxed state. If you find yourself judging, simply observe that too, and then let it go, coming back to your practice.

After you have been meditating for some time and you feel comfortable with the process, you may find that you experience a voice. Some say that they hear their "inner voice" or their "higher self." You may choose to ask a question or you may not. Perhaps you will hear words of wisdom or answers to questions you already have. Some people say that this inner dialogue comes naturally for them and is enlightening; others don't experience it at all. Whatever you experience is right for you.

HOW OFTEN TO MEDITATE

Meditation should be practiced as often as possible, with your goal being sessions of at least 20 minutes each day of the week. While you can meditate longer than 20 minutes, it is preferable that you meditate every day even if only for 10-minute sessions. Initially, it may take you a while to become completely relaxed and clear your mind of the mental chatter. However, as you become more experienced, you will attain this calm state more quickly. Ideally, you should set aside a specific time each day that you devote to meditation. Perhaps it will be early in the morning before work or school, in the middle of the day at your lunch hour, or just after you arrive home in the evening. At home, make a point of meditating in the same place so there won't be new distractions and adjustments to make with each meditation session.

Some other opportunities for learning to relax your body and mind and increase your awareness of the influence you have over your physical and emotional states include biofeedback training, yoga, and tai chi, which is actually a moving meditation.

AFTERWORD

At this point, we have completed the Whole Health Equation. As you have seen in these pages, and as many others are discovering, each of us can dramatically influence our own level of wellness. We have seen that nutrition can play a powerful role in the prevention of numerous chronic diseases, and that by choosing healthful foods and following the guidelines of the Revised American Diet, we can not only help prevent the onset of these diseases, but also boost our immunity and thereby reduce our susceptibility to various opportunistic illnesses, as well as experience more energy and easy weight management.

We have seen how important it is for each of us to maintain muscular flexibility, strength, and tone in order to assure proper physical function and maximum mobility well into our later years.

It has been shown that aerobic conditioning is not only essential to the maintenance of the heart, lungs, and blood vessels, but also can play an important role in weight management and boosting immunity, as well as preventing hypertension, adult-onset diabetes, osteoporosis, and many other conditions.

Finally, we have seen that in order to complete the equation and achieve maximum well-being, we should strive for greater mindfulness. Knowing that our thoughts and feelings can powerfully influence bodily functions, and thus either empower or impair our health, proves that exercising the mind is just as important as exercising the muscles, heart, and lungs.

Unfortunately, a large part of the medical community still has much catching up to do in regard to these truths. I am reminded of a simple story. A community was built upon a precipice, and, as a result, there were frequent accidents in which people fell, hurt themselves, and sometimes died. When the problem worsened, a meeting of the townspeople was called to determine what might be done to rectify the problem. On one side of the meeting room there were cries for funds so that an ambulance could be purchased and parked at the bottom of the precipice. That way, it was reasoned, when someone fell, they could be driven quickly to the hospital. On the other side, however, there was a request for funds to erect a simple fence around the precipice, thereby preventing the accidents from occurring in the first place.

We need more fence building and less reliance on treatment and curative approaches. You now have the knowledge to create healthy change – to erect your own preventive fence, so to speak. The sooner you begin to apply the principles of Whole Health to your life, the sooner you will begin to experience the many health benefits it offers.

I live the Whole Health lifestyle I am advocating in these pages, and there is rarely a day that passes that I do not consider the incredible health benefits I have enjoyed as a result of this lifestyle. While I used to fall prey to the "inevitable" cold or flu that seems to be a regular part of many people's lives, this is no longer the case for me. In fact, I cannot remember the last time I had a cold. Yet this benefit cannot be simply attributed to greater immune strength. By following the Revised American Diet, I have eliminated my exposure to a significant source of bacterial infection—animal products.

One of the most important dividends I have received from Whole Health living is a major drop in my cholesterol. Three years ago, my total cholesterol was determined to be 187 mg/dl. While this was below the national average for adults, which is 205 mg/dl, I wanted to reduce my risk even more. I set my sights on 150 mg/dl because this level has been determined to represent very little risk of heart disease. At the time of this writing I have just received the results of a recent blood panel, and, frankly, I am delighted. Not only have I reached my goal of 150 mg/dl, but I have far surpassed it, bringing my total cholesterol to only 116 mg/dl! Some may think me a bit strange sharing this "irrelevant" number with them as though it were a winning lottery number. Yet those who understand are very impressed and convinced that they too can create changes in their lifestyle that will reap them significant benefits.

I share this with you because I wish to reiterate that Whole Health is not a fad, it is not an illusive health gimmick in which promises are made and results are unattainable, and it is not armchair theory. By following the lifestyle I am advocating, I know for certain that you can attain similar health benefits.

By following the principles outlined in this book, you will nurture Whole Health for the rest of your life. But don't stop here. I hope you will continue to educate yourself about your body and mind. Seek out material by credible authors to keep yourself current on recent developments in the area of well-being, and help your friends and loved ones by sharing what you learn.

I wish you the best of health!

APPENDIX

MAGAZINES

Delicious!
1301 Spruce Street
Boulder, CO 80302
(302) 939-8440

Veggie Life
P.O. Box 57159
Boulder, CO 80322

Vegetarian Gourmet
P.O. Box 7641
Riverton, NJ 08077

Vegetarian Times
P.O. Box 570
Oak Park, IL 60303
(708) 848-8100

Organic Gardening
33 East Minore Street
Emmaus, PA 18098
(215) 967-8154

ENVIRONMENTAL ORGANIZATIONS

EarthSave
706 Frederick Street
Santa Cruz, CA 95062
(408) 423-4069

Rainforest Action Network (RAN)
450 Sansome Street, Suite 700
San Francisco, CA 94111
(415) 398-4404

Earth Island Institute
300 Broadway, Suite 28
San Francisco, CA 94133
(415) 788-3666

Organic Trade Association
P.O. Box 1078, 20 Federal Street, #3
Greenfield, MA 01302
(413) 774-7511

Natural Organic Farmer's Association
411 Sheldon Road
Barre, MA 01005
(508) 355-2853

Youth for Environmental Sanity
706 Frederick Street
Santa Cruz, CA 95062
(408) 459-9344

Vegan Action
P.O. Box 4353
Berkeley, CA 94704
(510) 654-6297
HTTP://www.Vegan.org

Multi-Pure Water Purification Systems
P.O. Box 4179
Chatsworth, CA 91313
(800) 622-9206

American Holistic Medical Association (AHMA)
4101 Lake Boone Trail, #201
Raleigh, NC 27607
(919) 787-5146

Physicians Committee for Responsible Medicine (PCRM)
5100 Wisconsin Avenue, Suite 404
Washington, D.C. 20016
(202) 686-2210

American Vegan Society
501 Old Harding Highway
Malaga, NJ 08328
(609) 694-2887

North American Vegetarian Society (NAVS)
P.O. Box 72
Dolgeville, NY 13329
(518) 568-7970

Transcendental Meditation Center Directory
(800) 843-8332

Biofeedback Therapy Directory
Biofeedback Certification Institute of America
10200 West 44th Avenue, Suite 304
Wheat Ridge, CO 80033
(303) 420-2902

Vegetarian Nutrition Dietetic Practice Group
American Dietetic Association
216 W. Jackson Boulevard
Chicago, IL 60606
(312) 899-0040

MIT Vegetarian Support Group
Massachusetts Institute of Technology
Cambridge, MA
HTTP://www.mit.edu:8001/
activities/vsg/home.html

Vegetarian Society of the United Kingdom
Parkdale, Dunham Road
Altrinchan, Cheshire
WA14 4QG England
(0161) 928-0793
Vegsoc@vegsoc.demon.co.uk.

GUIDE TO REGIONAL AND NATIONAL
HEALTH FOOD STORES AND SUPERMARKETS

Alfalfa's, *Denver, Vail, CO*

Amigo Natural Grocery, *Taos, NM*

Bread and Circus, *MA*

Cornucopia, *Northhampton, MA*

Erewhon Market, *Los Angeles, CA*

First Alternative, *Corvallis, OR*

Food for Thought, *Westport, CT*

Fresh Fields *(national)*

Good Food Store, *Missoula, MT*

Healthy You Market, *Marco Island, FL*

Mrs. Gooch's, *Los Angeles, CA*

Oasis Natural Grocery, *Ithaca, NY*

The Real Food Company, *CA*

Super Natural Foods, *Corte Madera, CA*

The Vitamin Cottage, *Denver, CO*

Weaver Street Market, *Carrboro, NC*

Wellspring Grocery, *Austin, TX*

Wild Oats Markets *(Western States)*

Whole Foods Markets *(national)*

Zucchini's, *Athens, GA*

NATURAL FOOD BRANDS

The following is a listing of natural, brand-name foods available at better natural foods markets, many of which are available organic. In the event that your favorite market does not carry these brands, present the manufacturer/distributor name to the market manager so that they may begin stocking the products.

BREAKFAST CEREALS

Nature's Path
Corn flakes
Raisin bran
Heritage (quinoa,
   kamut, spelt)
Multigrain

Nature's Path Foods, Inc.
7453 Progress Way
Delta, B.C. V4G 1E8

Health Valley
Healthy fiber (org)
Oatbran (org)
Amaranth flakes (org)
Bran

Health Valley Foods, Inc.
16100 Foothill Boulevard
Irwindale, CA 91706

Kashi Company
Kashi Medley
Puffed Kashi

Kashi Company
P.O. Box 8557
La Jolla, CA 92038

Pacific Grain Products
Nutty corn
Nutty rice
Nutty wheat

Pacific Grain Products, Inc.
P.O. Box 2060
Woodland, CA 95776

Arrowhead Mills
Bran flakes (org)
Kamut (org)
Spelt flakes (org)
Corn flakes (org)
Amaranth flakes (org)
Oat bran flakes (org)

Arrowhead Mills, Inc.
Hereford, TX 79045

NON-DAIRY MAYONNAISE AND SPREADS

Nayonaise

Nasoya Foods, Inc.
Leominister, MA 01453
(800) 229-8638

Vegenaise
Earth Island

Follow Your Heart
7848 Alabama Avenue
Canoga Park, CA
(818) 347-9946

Spectrum Spread
(butter replacement, free of
hydrogenated oils)

Spectrum Naturals, Inc.
133 Copeland Street
Petaluma, CA 94952

NON-DAIRY BEVERAGES

Vitasoy
"light" (1% fat, org)
original, cocoa, vanilla

Vitasoy USA
Brisbane, CA 94005
(800) VITASOY

Edensoy
Edensoy "extra"
(beta carotene, calcium, B$_{12}$
E & D fortified, org)

Eden Foods, Inc.
Clinton, MI 94236

Rice Dream
Rice dream enriched
(A, D, and calcium fortified)

Imagine Foods, Inc.
350 Cambridge Avenue, Suite 350
Palo Alto, CA 94306

Almond "Mylk"

Wholesome & Hearty Foods, Inc.
2422 S.E. Hawthorne Boulevard
Portland, OR 97214
(800) 636-0109

Westsoy
(calcium, A & D fortified, org)

Westbrae Natural Foods
Carson, CA 90746
(310) 886-8200

PANCAKE MIXES

Arrowhead Mills
Blue corn
Multi grain
Oat bran
Buckwheat
Gluten-free

Arrowhead Mills, Inc.
Hereford, TX 79045

FLOURS

Arrowhead Mills
Millet flour
Soy flour
Oat flour
Buckwheat flour
Barley flour
Kamut flour
Spelt flour

Arrowhead Mills, Inc.
Hereford, TX 79045

BREADS

Pacific Bakery
Kamut bread
Kamut bagels
Spelt bread
(all yeast-free)

Pacific Bakery
P.O. Box 950
Oceanside, CA 92049

Food For Life
Rice & Almond bread
Ener-G

Food For Life Baking Co.
2991 E. Doherty Street
Corona, CA 91719

Rudi's Bakery
100% rye
Whole grain

Rudi's Bakery
Boulder, CO 80301

NUT BUTTERS

Arrowhead Mills
Peanut butter
   ("sunshine dried",
   non-hydrogenated)

Arrowhead Mills, Inc.
Hereford, TX 79045

Maranatha Natural Foods
Almond butter (org)
Cashew butter
Sunflower butter
Sesame butter

Maranatha Natural Foods, Inc.
P.O. Box 1046
Ashland, OR 97520

Baughen Ranch Produce
Almond butter (org)

PASTA SAUCES

Muir Glen
(org)

Muir Glen
P.O. Box 1498
Sacramento, CA 95812

Millina's Finest (org)

Organic Food Products, Inc.
P.O. Box 1510
Freedom, CA 95019

Whole Foods (org)

Whole Foods Markets
Austin, TX 78703

Enrico's (org)

Ventre Packing Co.
Syracuse, NY 13204

Garden Valley (org)

Garden Valley Naturals
S & D Foods, Inc.
Burlingame, CA 94011

PASTA

Eden (org)　　　　　　　Eden Foods, Inc.
　　　　　　　　　　　　　Clinton, MI 94236

Tuterri's

Michelle's Natural
(org)

Vita Spelt　　　　　　　Purity Foods, Inc.
(org)　　　　　　　　　　　2871 W. Jolly Road
　　　　　　　　　　　　　Okemos, MI 48864

Ener-G Brand　　　　　　Ener-G Foods, Inc.
(rice pasta)　　　　　　　　P.O. Box 84487
　　　　　　　　　　　　　Seattle, WA 98124
　　　　　　　　　　　　　(800) 331-5222

Pastariso　　　　　　　　Pastariso Products, Inc.
(rice pasta)　　　　　　　　55 Ironside
　　　　　　　　　　　　　Units 6 & 7 Scarborough
　　　　　　　　　　　　　Ontario, Canada M1X 1N3

Quinoa　　　　　　　　　Quinoa Corporation
　　　　　　　　　　　　　P.O. Box 1039
　　　　　　　　　　　　　Torrance, CA 90505

Westbrae Natural Foods　Westbrae Natural Foods
　　　　　　　　　　　　　Carson, CA 90746
　　　　　　　　　　　　　(310) 886-8200

Eddie's Pasta　　　　　　Mrs. Leepers, Inc.
　　　　　　　　　　　　　Poway, CA 92064

Tree of Life　　　　　　　Tree of Life, Inc.
　　　　　　　　　　　　　St. Augustine, FL
　　　　　　　　　　　　　32085-0410

CHIPS

Guiltless Gourmet
(baked chips)

Guiltless Gourmet, Inc.
3709 Promontory Point Drive
Suite. 131
Austin, TX 78744

Bearitos Chips
(baked chips)

Little Bear Organic Foods
Carson, CA 90746

Barbara's All Natural Chips
(baked chips)

Barbara's Baking, Inc.
3900 Cypress Drive
Petaluma, CA 94954

Garden of Eatin'
(baked chips)

Garden of Eatin', Inc.
Los Angeles, CA 90029

SPICES

The Spice Hunter
(non-irradiated)

The Spice Hunter, Inc.
San Luis Obispo, CA 93401

Spice Garden
(non-irradiated)

Modern Products, Inc.
P.O. Box 09398
Milwaukee, WI 53209

VEGETARIAN COOKBOOKS

Fields of Greens, by Annie Somerville, Executive Chef, Greens Restaurant, San Francisco, Bantam Books

The American Vegetarian Cookbook from the Fit for Life Kitchen, by Harvey and Marilyn Diamond, Warner Books

The Cookbook for People Who Love Animals, Gentle World, Inc.

The High Road to Health, by Lindsay Wagner and Ariane Spade, Prentice Hall Press

The McDougall Plan Recipes, Volume One, by Mary McDougall, New Win Publishing, Inc.

The Peaceful Palate: Fine Vegetarian Cuisine, by Jennifer Raymond

The Vegan Kitchen, by Freya Dinshah, The American Vegan Society

New Vegetarian Food, by Christine McFadden, Macmillan Publishing Company

Ecological Cooking: Recipes to Save the Planet, by Joanne Stepaniak and Kathy Hecker, The
   Book Publishing Company

Friendly Foods, Gourmet Vegetarian Cuisine, by Brother Ron Pickarski, O.F.M, Ten Speed Press

Simply Vegan Quick Vegetarian Meals, by Debra Wasserman, The Vegetarian Resource Group

If you have had a positive experience from following the lifestyle changes presented in this
book, we would like to know about it. Please send your comments to:

WHOLE HEALTH

Parissound Publishing
16 Miller Avenue, Suite 203
Mill Valley, CA 94941 U.S.A.

Please include your name, address, and a telephone number where you can be contacted.

GLOSSARY OF TERMS

ADIPOSE TISSUE Scientific name for fat tissue.

AEROBIC EXERCISE Exercises that employ the large muscle groups and are performed in a rhythmic and continuous fashion, at moderate intensity, for a duration of 15 minutes or longer.

AMINO ACIDS A variety of compounds, some essential, that are the building blocks that form proteins. Over 20 amino acids occur in nature.

ANAEROBIC EXERCISE Exercise of high intensity and short duration. Anaerobic exercises exceed the body's aerobic capacity, creating an oxygen debt. An example is sprinting.

ANTIOXIDANTS Agents, natural, or synthetic, including but not limited to vitamins C and E, beta carotene, and selenium, that are used by the body to neutralize free radicals. In the absence of sufficient antioxidants, free-radical chain reactions can lead to the destruction of tissues and development of disease.

ATHEROSCLEROSIS Occurs when plaque composed of cholesterol and other components accumulates along the arterial walls, progressively narrowing the channel. As narrowing advances, blood supply to the heart, brain, muscles, and other organs is diminished. In severe cases, one or more arteries may become completely blocked by plaque, resulting in heart attack or stroke.

BARBELL The fundamental training apparatus in free-weight exercises, consisting of the bar, weights, sleeves, and collars. Some barbells are "fixed" with a certain poundage that cannot be altered. Others are classified as "Olympic," measuring six feet in length and allowing for an assortment of plates to be loaded and unloaded by the user.

BETA CAROTENE One of many plant pigments, beta carotene is the precursor of vitamin A and is believed to be an important antioxidant.

BLOOD PRESSURE The force of blood against the arterial walls, blood pressure is measured in millimeters of mercury. There are two phases measured, including *systolic* (force generated during the contraction of the heart) and *diastolic* (force measured during relaxation of the heart). Blood pressure is said to be high when the systolic (upper number) is 140 or higher, and the diastolic (lower number) is 90 or higher.

CARDIOVASCULAR Pertaining to the heart and blood vessels.

CHEATING Any swaying, jerking, bouncing, or other extraneous body movement used to coax a weight past a sticking point, or point at which the muscles would normally fail.

CIRCUIT TRAINING Specialized type of weight training that allows for aerobic conditioning. Normally, a circuit of exercise "stations" is set up in the gym. The individual moves from station to station with little or no rest between exercises, until the entire circuit has been completed.

COLLAR The securing ring that slides on to the end of barbells. Inside collars prevent the weight plates from sliding in toward the hands and outside collars prevent the plates from sliding off the ends of the barbell.

CONTRACTION The shortening and lengthening of the muscle fiber when performing an exercise (isotonic contraction) or when a muscle exerts a force against a static resistance (isometric contraction). There is no change in actual muscle length.

ECG Electrocardiogram. Monitoring and recording of the electrical activity of the heart. An ECG provides important information regarding excitation of the heart, cardiac rhythm, and myocardial damage.

FATTY ACID A carbon chain with hydrogen atoms attached and an acidic chemical group at one end. Fatty acids are classified by the lengths of the chain (from 4 to 26 or more) and by whether all available chemical bonds are occupied with hydrogen atoms. Unsaturated fatty acids have one (monounsaturated) or more (polyunsaturated) links in the chain with double or triple bonds between carbons. Saturated fatty acids have no double bonds in the carbon chain and all available positions are occupied with hydrogen.

FDA The U. S. Food and Drug Administration.

FIBER A non-caloric component found only in plants. There are two types of fiber: insoluble and soluble. Insoluble fiber is not soluble in water and is found in the plant cell walls. Examples include most seeds and whole grains. Soluble fiber dissolves in water, forming a gel solution. This type of fiber is found in vegetables, oat bran, dried beans, and the pulp of fruit.

FLEXIBILITY The degree to which muscles and joints allow for free and exaggerated range of motion.

FORCED REPS An advanced training technique that allows a muscle to be further taxed after having reached a point of temporary failure. Normally a spotter or partner will assist in the lift of a barbell or dumbbells, slightly reducing the weight load, until the exerciser has passed the point of muscle failure. Forced reps are usually performed during the last two to three reps of a set in an effort to increase muscle fiber recruitment and induce greater increases in muscular strength and endurance.

FREE RADICAL A highly reactive molecule containing an unpaired electron. Free radicals search for electrons from other non-radicals. In doing so, they may create other free radicals. The result can be a destructive chain reaction that leads to disease.

GLUCOSE The most important carbohydrate in metabolism, it is the primary source of energy. Excess glucose is stored as glycogen in the liver and muscles.

GLYCOGEN The form in which glucose is stored in the body for later use as fuel.

HEART RATE The number of heart beats per minute.

HYPERTENSION Hypertension exists at blood pressure levels of 140/90 millimeters of mercury and above. Ninety-five percent of hypertension cases are labeled "essential" or "idiopathic" because their cause is unknown. However, several risk factors are recognized, including a sodium-rich diet. Hypertension increases the risk for heart disease, stroke, and kidney failure.

HYPERTROPHY The increase in overall size of a muscle as a result of an increase in the size of the individual muscle fibers.

INSULIN A hormone secreted by the beta cells of the pancreas. Insulin production is dependent upon blood glucose levels. An increase in blood glucose will increase insulin production, which in turn stimulates the transport of glucose into cells.

INTENSITY The quality and degree of energy and strength applied to an exercise.

INUIT Those people native to Arctic America.

ISOLATION EXERCISE Exercise limiting the stress to a specific muscle or muscle group. Basic exercises employ larger as well as synergistic muscles and muscle groups.

KETONE Chemical substance that results from incomplete metabolism of fatty acids due to carbohydrate deficiency. Ketones occur most often with poorly managed diabetes, high-fat diets, and starvation.

LEAN BODY MASS Weight of the body minus fat content.

MASS Overall size of a muscle.

METABOLIC RATE The rate at which the body utilizes energy.

METABOLISM All chemical changes in an organism that support life.

NUTRITION The science of the intake and utilization of food substances for the purpose of maintaining good health.

OSSIFICATION Process whereby cartilage turns to bone.

OVERLOAD When a muscle is subjected to a resistance or weight load greater than it is accustomed.

POUNDAGE The actual weight being used as a resistance in any exercise.

PROGRAM Also known as a routine, the list of exercises and the repetitions, sets, and poundages used to perform them.

PROSTAGLANDIN Hormone-like substances that are derived from fatty acids. The human body may contain up to 90 different prostaglandins.

PUMP Temporary enlargement of a muscle or muscle group brought about by the congestion of blood.

REPETITION Also called a rep, the single movement performed in a set. Each time the muscle contracts against a resistance, a single repetition has been performed.

RESISTANCE The force applied to a muscle or muscle group by way of free weights, machines, or other training apparatuses, in an effort to increase muscle strength.

ROUTINE Same as program; the exercises, sets, reps, and poundages used in a workout.

SET A group of repetitions performed without rest.

TARGET HEART RATE A heart rate considered safe and effective for aerobic exercise.

TRAINING TO FAILURE Continuing to perform repetitions in an exercise until the muscles no longer permit a complete repetition without the assistance of a spotter or partner.

VALSALVA MANEUVER Exhaling forcefully with the mouth closed in a manner that traps air. This generates great pressure in the chest cavity, decreases blood return to the heart, and increases blood pressure. In extreme cases it will cause fainting.

VEGAN One who excludes all animal products from his or her diet.

WARM-UP Any light-intensity exercise or stretching that prepares the body for greater energy output. Proper warm-ups facilitate an increase in body temperature, muscle elasticity and contractility, and cardiovascular adaptations.

WEIGHT TRAINING Using barbells, dumbbells, machines, or other apparatuses to change the appearance and level of conditioning of the body.

NOTES

1   American Heart Association, *Heart and Stroke Facts* (1994).

2   American Heart Association, *Heart and Stroke Facts* (1994). Statistical Supplement.

3   American Dietetic Association, "Position of the American Dietetic Association: Vegetarian Diets," *Journal of the American Dietetic Association* 93 (1993):1317-19.

4   American Dietetic Association, "Position of the American Dietetic Association: Vegetarian diets" (technical support paper), *Journal of the American Dietetic Association* 88 (1988):352-54.

5   EarthSave Foundation, *Realities for the '90s* (1992),12.

6   Parr, R.B., et al. "Nutrition Knowledge and Practices of Coaches, Trainers, and Athletes," *Physician Sports Medicine* 12 (1984):127.

    Pratt, Charlotte A., et al., "Nutrition Knowledge and Concerns of Health and Physical Education Teachers," *Journal of the American Dietetic Association* 88 (1988):840-41.

7   Committee on Diet, Nutrition and Cancer, *Diet, Nutrition and Cancer* (Washington, D.C.: National Academy Press, 1982).

8   Willet, W.C., "Dietary Fat and Risk of Breast Cancer," *New England Journal of Medicine* 316 (1987):22-28.

9   *Prevention '82*, DHHS publication no. (PHS) 82-50157 (Washington, D.C.: Office of Disease Prevention and Health Promotion, 1982).

10 "The Good Doctor" "CBS Dateline" transcript. Interview with Dr. Susan Love. September 28, 1994, 14.

11 Richardson, Sylvia, "The Role of Fat, Animal Protein and Some Vitamin Consumption in Breast Cancer: A Case Control Study in Southern France," *International Journal of Cancer* 48 (1991):1-9.

12 EarthSave Foundation, *Realities for the '90s* (1992), 9.

13 Epstein, Samuel S. "The Chemical Jungle: Today's Beef Industry," *International Journal of Health Services* 20 (1990):277-80.

14 Colditz, Graham A., et al, "The Use of Estrogens and Progestins and the Risk of Breast Cancer in Postmenopausal Women," *New England Journal of Medicine* 332 (1995):1589-93.

15 EarthSave Foundation, *Realities for the '90s* (1992), 7.

16 Mott, Abraham M., *Your Daily Dose of Pesticide Residues*. (San Francisco: Pesticide Action Network International)

17 Robbins, John. *Diet for a New America* (New Hampshire: Stillpoint,1987), 344.

18 Ibid., 345.

19 Hergenrather, J., et al., "Pollutants in Breast Milk of Vegetarians," *Lancet* 304 (1981): 792

20 "Red Meat Linked to Fatal Prostate Cancer," *San Francisco Chronicle*, 6 October 1993, sec. A4.

21 "Comparative Epidemiology of Cancers of the Colon, Rectum, Prostate and Breast in Shanghai, China, versus the United States," *International Journal of Epidemiology*, 20 (1991): 76-81.

22 Epstein, Samuel S., "The Chemical Jungle: Today's Beef Industry," *International Journal of Health Services* 20 (1990):277-80.

23 "Comparative Epidemiology of Cancers of the Colon, Rectum, Prostate and Breast in Shanghai, China, versus the United States." *International Journal of Epidemiology*, 20 (1991): 76-81.

24 Howell, Margaret A.,"Diet as an Etiological Factor in the Development of Cancers of the Colon and Rectum," *Journal of Chronic Disease* 28 (1975):67-80.

    Willet, Walter C., "Relation of Meat, Fat, and Fiber Intake to the Risk of Colon Cancer in a Prospective Study Among Women," *New England Journal of Medicine* 24 (1990):1664-71.

25 Feinleib, Manning, "The Magnitude and Nature of the Decrease in Coronary Heart Disease Mortality Rate," *The American Journal of Cardiology* 54 (1984): 2-5C.

26 EarthSave Foundation, *Realities for the '90s* (1992), 7.

27 Ibid., 8.

28 American Heart Association, *Heart and Stroke Facts* (1994)

29 Ibid., 20.

30 Ibid., 16.

31 Ibid., 1.

32 Lees, A.M., et al., "Plant Sterols as Cholesterol-lowering Agents: Clinical Trials in Patients with Hypercholesterolemia and Studies of Sterol Balance," *Atherosclerosis* 28 (1977):325-38.

33 American Heart Association, *Heart and Stroke Facts* (1994). Statistical Supplement.

34 Ibid.

35 John Hopkins Medical letter, *Health After 50* 8 (1996): 1

Merrill F., et al., "Untreated Blood Pressure Is Inversely Related to Cognitive Function: The Frammingham Study," *American Journal of Epidemiology* 138 (1993): 353-64.

36 Aronson, Virginia, et al., *Guidebook for Nutritional Counselors* (Prentice Hall, 1990), 111.

Margen, S., et al., "Studies in Calcium Metabolism: The Calciuretic Effect of Dietary Protein," *American Journal of Clinical Nutrition* 27 (1974): 584-9.

Licata, A., "Acute Effects of Increased Meat Protein on Urinary Electrolytes and Cyclic Adenosine Monophosphate and Serum Parathyroid Hormone," *American Journal of Clinical Nutrition* 34 (1981): 1779-84.

37 Abelow, Benjamin J, et al., "Cross-Cultural Association Between Dietary Animal Protein and Hip Fracture: A Hypothesis," *Calcified Tissue International* 50 (1992): 14-18.

"Calcium Supplementation of the Diet—I: Not Justified by Present Evidence," *British Medical Journal* 298 (1989): 137-40.

Lindsay, H., et al., "Protein-induced Hypercalciuria: A Longer Term Study," *American Journal of Clinical Nutrition* 32 (1979): 741-49.

"How Important is Dietary Calcium?," *Science* 233 (1986): 519-20.

38 Marsh, A.G., et al., "Vegetarian Lifestyle and Bone Mineral Density," *American Journal of Clinical Nutrition* 48 (1988):837-41.

39 Walker, A., "The Influence of Numerous Pregnancies and Lactations on Bone Dimensions in South African Bantu and Caucasian Mothers," *Clinical Science* 42 (1972): 189-196.

40 U.S. Department of Agriculture, "Nutrition and Your Health: Dietary Guidelines for Americans" (1996):8.

41 Leaf, Alexander, "Cardiovascular Effects of n-3 Fatty Acids," *New England Journal of Medicine* 318 (1988): 549-57.

42 Phillipson, B.E., et al., "Reduction of Plasma Lipids, Lipoproteins, and Apoproteins by Dietary Fish Oils in Patients with Hypertriglyceridemia," *New England Journal of Medicine* 312 (1985): 1210-16.

43 Howard, Barbara V., et al., "Polyunsaturated Fatty Acids Result in Greater Cholesterol Lowering and Less Triacylglycerol Elevation than Do Monounsaturated Fatty Acids in a Dose Response Comparison in a Multiracial Study Group," *The American Journal of Clinical Nutrition* 62 (1995): 392-402.

44 Erasmus, Udo. *Fats and Oils* (Alive Books, 1986), 111.

Schaefer, Ernst J., et al., "Lipoproteins, Nutrition, Aging and Atherosclerosis," *American Journal of Clinical Nutrition* 61 (1995): 726s-740s.

45 Erasmus, Udo. *Fats and Oils* (Alive Books, 1986), 111.

46 Willet, W.C., et al. "Intake of Fatty Acids and Risk of Coronary Heart Disease Among Women," *The Lancet* 341 (1993):581-85.

47   Westrate, Jan A., et al., "Sucrose Polyester and Plasma Carotenoid Concentrations in Healthy Subjects," *American Journal of Clinical Nutrition* 62 (1995): 591-7.

48   Cunnane, Steven C., et al., "Nutritional Attributes of Traditional Flaxseed in Healthy Young Adults" *American Journal of Clinical Nutrition* 61 (1995): 62-8.

49   Kelley, D.S., et al., "Dietary Alpha-linolenic Acid and Immunocompetence in Humans" *American Journal of Clinical Nutrition* 53 (1991): 40-6.

Marshall, L.A., et al., "The Effect of Alpha-linolenic Acid in the Rat on Fatty Acid Profiles of Immunocompetent Cell Populations" *Lipids* 18 (1983): 737-42.

50   Bierenbaum M.L., et al., "Reducing Atherogenic Risk in Hyperlipemic Humans with Flaxseed Supplementation: A Preliminary Report" *Journal of the American College of Nutrition* 12 (1993): 501-4.

51   Kaiser, John D., *Immune Power* (New York: St. Martin's Press, 1993), 26.

52   Larson, David E., *Mayo Clinic Family Health Book* (New York: William Morrow and Company, 1990), 330.

53   Garrett, Laurie, *The Coming Plague* (New York: Farrar, Straus and Giroux, 1994), 42.

54   U. S. Environmental Protection Agency, *Environmental News*, 11 May 1993.

55   *Delicious* (April 1995):38.

56   Fox, Martin, *Healthy Water* (Portsmouth: Healthy Water Research, 1990), 12.

57   Weininger, Jean, *San Francisco Chronicle*, 6 October, sec. F.1.

58   Wigle, D.T., et al., "Contaminants in Drinking Water and Cancer in Canadian Cities," *Canadian Journal of Public Health* 77 (1986):335-41.

59   *USA Today* 18-20 February 1994.

60   *The Mayo Clinic Family Health Book* (New York: William Morrow and Company, 1990),330.

61   *San Francisco Chronicle*, 2 February 1994, sec. A6.

62   Byers, T., et al., "Epidemiologic Evidence for Vitamin C and Vitamin E in Cancer Prevention," *American Journal of Clinical Nutrition* 62 (1995 Suppl):1385S-92S.

63   Block, G., "Vitamin C and Cancer Prevention: the Epidemiologic Evidence," *American Journal of Clinical Nutrition* 53 (1991 Suppl): 270S-83S.

Byers, T., et al., "Dietary Carotenes, Vitamin C, and Vitamin E as Protective Antioxidants in Human Cancers," *Annual Reviews of Nutrition* 12 (1992): 139-59.

University of California Berkeley Wellness Letter 10, 4 (January 1994).

64   Enstrom, J.E., et al., *Epidemiology* 3 (1992):194-202.

Kohlmeier, L., et al., "Epidemiologic Evidence of a Role of Carotenoids in Cardiovascular Disease Prevention," *American Journal of Clinical Nutrition* 62 (1995 Suppl): 1370S-6S.

Jaques, P.F., et al., "Epidemiologic Evidence of a Role for the Antioxidant Vitamins and Carotenoids in Cataract Prevention," *American Journal of Clinical Nutrition* 53 (1991):352S-55S.

65   Meydani, S., et al., "Vitamin E Supplementation Enhances Cell-mediated Immunity in Healthy Elderly Subjects," *American Journal of Clinical Nutrition* 52 (1990):557-63.

66   Buring, J.E., et al., *Cancer Prevention* 89 (July 1989).

67   Newberne, P.M., et al., "Nutrition and Cancer: A Review with Emphasis on the Role of Vitamins C and E and Selenium," *Nutrition and Cancer* 5 (1983):107-19.

68   Olanow, C.W., "An Introduction to the Free Radical Hypothesis in Parkinson's Disease," *Annals of Neurology* 32 (1992):S2-S9.

69   Sanders, T.A.B., et al., "Haematological Studies on Vegans," *British Journal of Nutrition* 40 (1978): 9-15.

70   Carlson, E., et al., "A Comparative Evaluation of Vegan, Vegetarian and Omnivore Diets," *Journal of Plant Foods* 6 (1985): 89-100.

71   Ruskin, A., *Classics in Arterial Hypertension* (Springfield, MA: Charles C. Thomas, 1956).

72   Epstein, Samuel S. "The Chemical Jungle: Today's Beef Industry," *International Journal of Health Services* 20 (1990):277-80.

73   Ibid.

74   Hirayama, T. Paper presented at the conference on Breast Cancer and Diet. U.S.-Japan Cooperative Cancer Research Program, Fred Hutchinson Center, Seattle, WA. 14-15 March 1977.

75   Rashmi, Sinha, et al., *Cancer Research* 54 (1994): 6154-59.

Nagao, Minako, "Carcinogenic Factors in Food with Relevance to Colon Cancer Development." *Mutation Research* 290 (1993): 43-51.

76   "Is Your Food Safe?" CBS News 48 Hours transcript. (Burrelle's Information Services, New Jersey, 2 March, 1994) 20-2.

77   "Something Smells Fowl," *Time* 17 (October 1994): 42.

78   Clarkson, Thomas, "Environmental Contaminants in the Food Chain," *The American Journal of Clinical Nutrition* 61 (1995): 682s-686s.

79   Ibid.

80   Willet, Walter C., et al., "Galactose Consumption and Metabolism in Relation to the Risk of Ovarian Cancer," *The Lancet* 7 (1989):66-71.

Cramer, D.W., et al. "Characteristics of Women with a Family History of Ovarian Cancer, Galactose Consumption and Metabolism," *Cancer* 74 (1994): 1309-17.

81   Jukka, Karjalainen, et al., "A Bovine Albumin Peptide as a Possible Trigger of Insulin-dependent Diabetes Mellitus," *New England Journal of Medicine* July 30 (1992):302-7.

Work Group on Cow's Milk Protein and Diabetes Mellitus, American Academy of Pediatrics, "Infant Feeding Practices and Their Possible Relationship to the Etiology of Diabetes Mellitus," *Pediatrics* 94 (1994):752-54.

82   Epstein, Samuel, "Potential Public Health Hazards of Biosynthetic Milk Hormones," *International Journal of Health Services* 20 (1990): 73-84.

83   "Investigator's Report," *FDA Journal* 30 (1996): 34.

84   Sacks, F., "Ingestion of Egg Raises Plasma Low Density Lipoproteins in Free Living Subjects," *The Lancet* 1 (1984):647.

85   Brown, Judith E., *The Science of Human Nutrition* (New York: Harcourt Brace Jovanovich, 1990), 237.

86   *Journal of The American Medical Association*(JAMA) 274 (1995): 1328-30.

87   Krinsky, Norman, "The Evidence for the Role of Carotenoids in Preventive Health," *Clinical Nutrition* 7 (1988):107-12.

88   Anderson, James W., et al., "Meta-Analysis of the Effects of Soy Protein Intake On Serum Lipids," *New England Journal Of Medicine* 333 (1995): 276-82.

89   Kaiser, John D., *Immune Power* (New York: St. Martin's Press, 1993), 28-30.

90   Ibid.

91   Crocco, S.C., "The Role of Sodium in Food Processing," *Journal of the American Dietetic Association* 80 (1982):36-38.

92   Shank, F.R., et al., "Perspective of the Food and Drug Administration on Dietary Sodium," *Journal of the American Dietetic Association* 80 (1982):29-35.

93   Perlmutter, David, *LifeGuide* (Naples, FL: LG Press, 1992), 16.

94   Smith, C., S. Beckman, "Export of Pesticides from U.S. Ports in 1990: Focus on Restricted Pesticide Exports," *A Report to the Committee on Agriculture in Science and Education* 20 (Sept. 1991).

95   "Is Your Food Safe?" transcript, CBS News, 48 Hours. (Burrelle's Information Services, 20 March 1994),18.

Environmental Working Group, "Washed, Peeled—Contaminated," EWG (1994), Washington, D.C.

96   Mott, Abraham, M., *Your Daily Dose of Pesticide Residues* (San Francisco: Pesticide Action Network International, 1989).

97   Kaiser, John D., *Immune Power* (New York:, St. Martin's Press, 1993), 27.

98   Rowe, K.S., and K.J. Rowe, "Synthetic Food Coloring and Behavior: A Dose Response Effect in a Double-blind, Placebo-controlled, Repeated-measures Study," *Journal of Pediatrics* 125 (1994): 691-98.

99   Clyne, Patrick S., et al., "Human Breast Milk Contains Bovine IgG. Relationship to Infant Colic?" *Pediatrics* 87 (1991): 439-43.

100   Ziegler, E.E., et al., "Cow Milk Feeding in Infancy: Further Observations on Blood Loss From the Gastrointestinal Tract," *Journal of Pediatrics* 116 (1990):11-18.

101   Lovendale, Mark, "The Impact of Dairy Products on Human Health, the Environment and the National Budget," *Advanced Health Journal* 5 (1993):1-12.

102   R. Coombs, S., et al., "Hypersensitivity to Milk and Sudden Death in Infancy," *The Lancet* 2 (1960).

      Coombs, R.R.A.,"Allergy and Cot Death: With Special Focus on Allergic Sensitivity to Cows' Milk and Anaphylaxis," *Clinical and Experimental Allergy* (20 July 1990):359-66.

103   Kagawa, Y. "Impact of Westernization of the Nutrition of Japanese: Changes in Physique, Cancer, Longevity and Centenarians," *Preventive Medicine* 7 (1978):205-17.

104   "Buffing Up Makes Old Bones Stronger," *San Francisco Chronicle*, 28 Dec. 1994, sec. A:5.

      Aloia J., "Prevention of Involutional Bone Loss by Exercise," *Annals of Internal Medicine* 89 (1978): 356-58

105   American Council on Exercise, *The Personal Trainer's Manual* (San Diego: ACE, 1991).

106   Ornish, Dean. "Can Lifestyle Changes Reverse Coronary Heart Disease?," *The Lancet* 336 (1990):129-33.

107   Final Report of the Subcommittee on Non-pharmacological Therapy of the 1984 Joint National Committee on Detection, Evaluation, and Treatment of High Blood Pressure, "Non Pharmacological Approaches to the Control of High Blood Pressure," *Hypertension* 8 (1986):444-60.

108   Barnard, R.J., et al., "Diet and Exercise in the Treatment of NIDDM: The Need for Early Emphasis," *Diabetes Care* 17 (1994):1469-72.

109   Justice, Blair, *Who Gets Sick* (Los Angeles: Jeremy P. Tarcher, Inc., 1987), 158.

110   Chopra, Deepak, *Ageless Body, Timeless Mind* (New York: Harmony Books, 1993), 23.

111   Kaplan, Kenneth H., et al., "The Impact of a Meditation-Based Stress Reduction Program on Fibromyalgia," *General Hospital Psychiatry* 15 (1993):284-89.

112   Cooper, Michael J., et al., "A Relaxation Technique in the Management of Hypercholesterolemia," *Journal of Human Stress* (Dec. 1979).

      Kabat-Zinn, John. "An Outpatient Program in Behavioral Medicine for Chronic Pain Patients Based on the Practice of Mindful Meditation: Theoretical Considerations and Preliminary Results," *General Hospital Psychiatry* 4 (1982):33-47.

113   Chopra, Deepak, *Ageless Body, Timeless Mind* (New York: Harmony Books, 1993), 165.

114   Ornish, Dean, et al., "Can Lifestyle Changes Reverse Coronary Heart Disease?" *The Lancet* 336 (1990):129-33.

INDEX

PCBs, 34, 117
Pesticides, 34, 140-143
Phosphorus, in cow's milk, 121
Physical exams, 223
Phytochemicals, 129
Polyunsaturated fat, 70
Progressive resistance exercise, 230-232
Prostaglandins, 68
Protein, 61-67
Pregnancy, and the RAD, 156-158
Pulse, *see* heart rate
Pyramid sets, 314
Resistance, 230, 284
Rest, 283
Running program, 272-275
Salmonella, 117
Salt, *see* sodium
Saturated fats, 69
Seeds, 134
Shoulders, exercises for, 340-344
Sodium,
    content of selected foods, 109
    hidden sources of, 110
Soreness, muscular, 287
Soups, 199-205
Soy foods, 131-133
Split routines, 294
Spotting, 295
Stress, defined, 379
    management of, 389-398
    and immune function, 382
Stretching, 237-248
Stripping, 310
Stroke, 41
Sugar, 136-138
Sudden infant death syndrome (SIDS), 153
Supersets, 312-313
Supplements, need for, 97-99
Talk test, 269

Target heart rate, 266-268
Tension-release method, 409-411
Time management, 399-401
Tofu, 131
Trans-fatty acids, 70-71
Triceps, exercises for, 360-364
    illustrated, 217
Trisets, 313-314
Valsalva maneuver, 287, 447
Vegetables, 128-131
Vegetarians, famous, 20-21
Very low density lipoprotein, 44
Visualization, 413-419
Vitamins, 91-101
Walking program, 271-272
Water, 82-89
Weight loss, 105-108
Women's concerns, 233-236

ORDER FORM

FAX ORDERS:
(415) 381-5374

TELEPHONE ORDERS:
(415) 383-2884/(888) 544-LIFE
Have Visa/Mastercard number ready.

MAIL ORDERS:
Parissound Publishing
16 Miller Avenue, Suite 203
Mill Valley, CA 94941 USA

NAME

ADDRESS

CITY   STATE   ZIP CODE

PHONE (   )

PAYMENT *(CHECK ONE)*:
☐ *CHECK*   ☐ *VISA*   ☐ *MASTERCARD*

CARD NUMBER:

NAME ON CARD: EXP. DATE:

SIGNATURE:

	PRICE:	QUANTITY:	AMOUNT:
	$24.00	X	
BOOK RATE: (3-4 WEEKS)	SHIPPING & HANDLING (SEE RATES TO THE LEFT)		
$3.50 for the first book,			
$1.25 for each additional book.	SUBTOTAL		
AIR MAIL:	SALES TAX (ADD 7.25% IN CA)		
$4.75 per book	TOTAL		

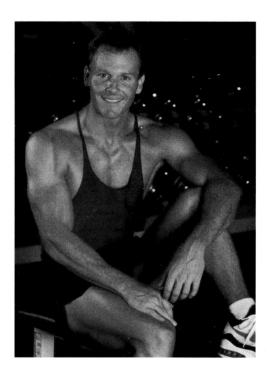

About the Author

Joseph Keon has been fascinated by the fitness and nutrition fields since the age of 14, when he discovered an abandoned weight set in the back of the family garage.

Starting with the time he first brought his high school class mates home to share his weights and insights, Joseph has continually refined his natural teaching skills. A fitness consultant for fifteen years, he continues to impress those who work with him by the depth of his knowledge and the ease with which he articulates that information.

Joseph received his *Physical Fitness Specialist* certification from Kenneth Cooper's Institute for Aerobic Research, is certified by the American Council on Exercise (ACE) and holds a Ph.D. in nutrition. He makes his home in Mill Valley, California.

In memory of Linda Sobek, whose grace
and professionalism made a significant
contribution to this project and
countless others.